PEJMAN HAJBABAIE

Understanding Metabolic Syndrome

First edition

This book was professionally typeset on Reedsy.
Find out more at reedsy.com

Contents

1

Chapter 1: Understanding Metabolic Syndrome

What Is Metabolic Syndrome?

Metabolic syndrome is a cluster of conditions that increase the risk of heart disease, stroke, and diabetes. It is characterised by a combination of high blood pressure, elevated blood sugar levels, excess body fat around the waist, and abnormal cholesterol levels. Understanding this syndrome is essential, as it affects a significant number of individuals globally and can lead to severe health complications if left unaddressed.

The prevalence of metabolic syndrome has been rising in recent years, largely due to lifestyle changes such as poor diet and physical inactivity. Many people are unaware that they may be living with this condition, as its symptoms can often be subtle or non-existent. Regular health screenings and awareness of the risk factors are crucial in identifying and managing metabolic syndrome in its early stages.

A critical aspect of managing metabolic syndrome involves lifestyle modifications. Adopting a balanced diet rich in whole grains, fruits, and vegetables, along with regular physical activity, can significantly improve health outcomes. Losing weight, if overweight, can also help to reduce the risk of developing associated diseases, making it a vital step for those affected.

In addition to lifestyle changes, medical intervention may be necessary for some individuals. Healthcare professionals may prescribe medications to help manage blood pressure, cholesterol, and blood sugar levels. Regular consultations with healthcare providers can ensure that individuals receive tailored advice and support in managing their metabolic health effectively.

Awareness and education about metabolic syndrome are paramount in combatting its impact on public health. By understanding what constitutes this syndrome and its potential risks, individuals can take proactive steps towards prevention and management. Initiatives aimed at increasing public knowledge and promoting healthier lifestyles can play a significant role in reducing the prevalence of metabolic syndrome in society.

Diagnostic Criteria (Waist circumference, BP, lipids, glucose)

The diagnostic criteria for metabolic syndrome focus on several key health indicators, including waist circumference, blood pressure, lipid levels, and glucose levels. Waist circumference is an important measure as it reflects central obesity, which is a significant risk factor for various metabolic disorders. For men, a waist measurement of more than 102 cm (40 inches) and for women, more than 88 cm (35 inches) indicates a higher risk of developing metabolic syndrome. This measurement is critical as it helps identify individuals who may be at increased risk even if their overall body weight appears normal.

Blood pressure is another essential component in diagnosing metabolic syndrome. Elevated blood pressure, defined as a reading of 130/85 mmHg or higher, can lead to serious cardiovascular issues. It is crucial to regularly monitor blood pressure as part of a comprehensive health assessment. Maintaining optimal blood pressure levels is essential for preventing complications associated with metabolic syndrome, such as heart disease and stroke.

Lipid levels, specifically triglycerides and HDL cholesterol, are key indicators of metabolic health. A triglyceride level of 150 mg/dL or higher, combined with an HDL cholesterol level of less than 40 mg/dL for men and less than 50 mg/dL for women, contributes to the diagnosis of metabolic syndrome. These lipid abnormalities are often linked to insulin resistance and can significantly increase the risk of cardiovascular disease.

Glucose levels also play a vital role in diagnosing metabolic syndrome. A fasting glucose level of 100 mg/dL or higher is indicative of impaired glucose metabolism, which is a fundamental aspect of metabolic syndrome. Regular glucose monitoring is essential, especially for those with other risk factors, as it can help in early detection and management of potential health issues.

In summary, the diagnostic criteria for metabolic syndrome encompass a combination of waist circumference, blood pressure, lipid levels, and glucose levels. Each of these factors contributes to a comprehensive assessment of an individual's metabolic health. By understanding and monitoring these criteria, individuals can take proactive steps towards reducing their risk of developing serious health conditions associated with metabolic syndrome.

Why It Matters: Long-Term Health Risks

Metabolic syndrome represents a cluster of conditions that significantly increase the risk of developing serious health issues over time. Understanding the long-term health risks associated with this syndrome is crucial for proactive management and prevention. Individuals with metabolic syndrome are often at a heightened risk for cardiovascular diseases, type 2 diabetes, and other chronic health problems that can ultimately diminish their quality of life. This awareness empowers individuals to make informed lifestyle choices and seek appropriate medical interventions to mitigate these risks.

One of the primary concerns linked to metabolic syndrome is its strong association with cardiovascular disease. The presence of high blood pressure, elevated blood sugar levels, and abnormal cholesterol can lead to plaque buildup in the arteries, resulting in heart attacks and strokes. Recognising these risks is essential not only for those diagnosed with metabolic syndrome but also for their families and communities, as the repercussions of cardiovascular disease extend far beyond the individual.

Moreover, individuals with metabolic syndrome are particularly vulnerable to developing type 2 diabetes. The interplay between obesity, insulin resistance, and metabolic abnormalities creates a perfect storm that can lead to this chronic condition. Understanding this connection can motivate individuals to adopt healthier eating habits and engage in regular physical activity, ultimately reducing their risk of diabetes and its associated complications, such as neuropathy and kidney damage.

The long-term health implications of metabolic syndrome also encompass mental health concerns. The stress of managing chronic physical health issues can lead to anxiety and depression, creating a vicious cycle that further exacerbates physical health problems. By addressing both the physical and mental health aspects of metabolic syndrome, individuals can foster a more holistic approach to their well-being, which is vital for a healthier future.

In conclusion, recognising the long-term health risks associated with metabolic syndrome is of paramount importance. By understanding these risks, individuals can take proactive steps towards prevention and management, leading to improved health outcomes. The journey towards better health is not solely about addressing one condition but involves a comprehensive understanding of how interconnected our physical and mental health truly is.

How It Develops Over Time

Metabolic syndrome is a complex condition that develops gradually over time, influenced by a multitude of factors including genetics, lifestyle, and environmental elements. Initially, individuals may not exhibit any noticeable symptoms, but subtle changes in body composition and metabolic processes are already underway. This stage often entails the accumulation of visceral fat and insulin resistance, which can lead to further complications if not addressed early on.

As time progresses, the effects of metabolic syndrome become more pronounced. Individuals may start to experience increased blood pressure, elevated cholesterol levels, and fluctuations in glucose metabolism. These changes are often insidious, making it challenging for individuals to recognise the seriousness of their condition until more significant health issues arise.

This progression underscores the importance of regular health screenings and awareness of one's metabolic health.

The development of metabolic syndrome is frequently linked to lifestyle choices such as diet and physical activity. Poor dietary habits, characterised by high sugar and fat intake, coupled with a sedentary lifestyle, can exacerbate the condition. Over time, these choices contribute to the worsening of metabolic markers, making it crucial for individuals to adopt healthier habits early in life to mitigate the risks associated with metabolic syndrome.

Moreover, psychological factors such as stress and lack of sleep can also play a significant role in the development of metabolic syndrome. Chronic stress can lead to hormonal imbalances that affect metabolism, while insufficient sleep can disrupt the body's ability to regulate insulin and glucose levels. Recognising the interplay between mental and physical health is vital in understanding how metabolic syndrome develops over time.

Ultimately, the trajectory of metabolic syndrome can be altered through proactive measures. Early intervention, including lifestyle modifications and medical management, can significantly improve outcomes and prevent the progression of the syndrome. By fostering a greater understanding of how metabolic syndrome develops, individuals can take charge of their health and work towards a healthier future.

2

Chapter 2: The Underlying Causes of Metabolic Syndrome

Insulin Resistance: The Core Problem

Insulin resistance is a condition that has become increasingly prevalent in modern society, contributing significantly to the rising rates of metabolic syndrome. This condition occurs when the body's cells become less responsive to insulin, a hormone crucial for regulating blood sugar levels. As a result, the pancreas compensates by producing more insulin, leading to a cycle that can ultimately result in higher blood sugar levels and an increased risk of type 2 diabetes.

The core problem of insulin resistance lies in its ability to disrupt normal metabolic processes. When cells fail to respond effectively to insulin, glucose remains in the bloodstream instead of being absorbed by the cells for energy. This not only elevates blood sugar levels but also forces the body to store excess fat, particularly in the abdominal region. This accumulation of visceral fat is particularly concerning, as it is associated with a range of health issues beyond diabetes, including cardiovascular disease and certain types of cancer.

Several factors contribute to the development of insulin resistance, including genetics, diet, and lifestyle choices. A diet high in refined carbohydrates and sugars can exacerbate the issue, as it leads to repeated spikes in blood sugar and insulin levels. Additionally, sedentary behaviour and obesity are significant risk factors, as excess body fat, especially around the abdomen, is known to impair insulin function. Understanding these contributors is crucial for managing and preventing insulin resistance.

Addressing insulin resistance requires a multifaceted approach that includes dietary changes, increased physical activity, and weight management. A balanced diet rich in whole foods, such as vegetables, lean proteins, and healthy fats, can help stabilise blood sugar levels and improve insulin sensitivity. Regular exercise not only helps in weight loss but also enhances the body's ability to use insulin effectively. For many, making these lifestyle changes can lead to significant improvements in metabolic health.

In conclusion, insulin resistance is a fundamental issue that underpins metabolic syndrome and poses serious health risks. Recognising the signs and understanding the mechanisms behind this condition is vital for individuals and healthcare providers alike. By prioritising lifestyle changes and addressing the factors that contribute to insulin resistance, it is possible to mitigate its effects and improve overall health outcomes.

Visceral Fat and Inflammation

Visceral fat, often referred to as abdominal or deep fat, is located around internal organs such as the liver, pancreas, and intestines. Unlike subcutaneous fat, which is found just beneath the skin, visceral fat poses a greater risk to health due to its proximity to vital organs. This type of fat is not only a storage site for excess energy but also an active endocrine organ that can release various inflammatory markers into the bloodstream.

The presence of excess visceral fat is closely linked to chronic inflammation in the body. When visceral fat cells expand, they can become dysfunctional and start producing pro-inflammatory cytokines. These substances can lead to a cascade of immune responses that contribute to the development of metabolic syndrome, a cluster of conditions that increase the risk of heart disease, stroke, and diabetes.

Chronic inflammation associated with visceral fat can disrupt the normal functioning of insulin, leading to insulin resistance. This condition is a major component of metabolic syndrome, where the body becomes less responsive to insulin, resulting in higher blood sugar levels. Over time, this can lead to type 2 diabetes, which further exacerbates the inflammatory state within the body.

Reducing visceral fat through lifestyle changes such as diet and exercise can significantly lower inflammation levels. Incorporating anti-inflammatory foods, regular physical activity, and stress management techniques can not only help reduce visceral fat but also improve overall metabolic health. These changes can foster a healthier environment within the body, mitigating the risks associated with metabolic syndrome.

Understanding the relationship between visceral fat and inflammation is vital for anyone aiming to improve their health. By recognising the detrimental effects of excess visceral fat, individuals can take proactive steps to reduce it and, in turn, lower inflammation. This holistic approach is essential for managing and potentially reversing the effects of metabolic syndrome, paving the way for a healthier future.

The Role of Genetics and Family History

Genetics play a significant role in the development of metabolic syndrome, influencing various risk factors such as obesity, insulin resistance, and dyslipidaemia. Individuals with a family history of metabolic disorders are often more susceptible to these conditions due to inherited genetic traits. Understanding the genetic predisposition can help identify those at risk and enable proactive measures to mitigate the onset of metabolic syndrome.

Family history is a crucial element in assessing an individual's risk for metabolic syndrome. When multiple family members have experienced issues related to obesity or diabetes, it raises the likelihood that genetic factors may be at play. This familial connection underscores the importance of gathering comprehensive health histories when evaluating personal health risks.

Moreover, epigenetics, which examines how environmental factors can influence gene expression, adds another layer of complexity to the discussion. Lifestyle choices such as diet, physical activity, and stress management can either exacerbate or alleviate genetic predispositions. Understanding this interplay helps individuals make informed decisions about their health.

Preventative strategies can be tailored based on genetic and family history insights. Individuals with a strong familial connection to metabolic syndrome may benefit from regular health screenings and lifestyle modifications aimed at reducing their risk. Educating families about their genetic background can promote a proactive approach to health and wellness.

In conclusion, the role of genetics and family history in metabolic syndrome is profound, impacting risk assessment and management strategies. By recognising these factors, individuals can take charge of their health and work towards preventing the onset of metabolic disorders. Awareness and education about genetic influences are vital in fostering healthier lifestyles within families.

Hormonal Imbalance (Leptin, Cortisol, Ghrelin)

Hormonal imbalance plays a significant role in the development and exacerbation of metabolic syndrome, particularly through the actions of leptin, cortisol, and ghrelin. Leptin, known as the "satiety hormone," is produced by adipose tissues and helps regulate energy balance by inhibiting hunger. However, in cases of obesity, leptin resistance can occur, leading to increased appetite and weight gain, which further complicates metabolic disorders. Understanding the dynamics of leptin is crucial for managing conditions associated with metabolic syndrome.

Cortisol, often referred to as the stress hormone, is another critical player in hormonal balance. It is released by the adrenal glands in response to stress and low blood glucose levels. While cortisol is essential for various bodily functions, chronic elevation due to prolonged stress can lead to increased fat accumulation, particularly in the abdominal area. This visceral fat is closely linked to the risks associated with metabolic syndrome, highlighting the need for stress management strategies.

Ghrelin, known as the "hunger hormone," is produced primarily in the stomach and stimulates appetite, promoting food intake and fat storage. Elevated levels of ghrelin can contribute to overeating and obesity, which are significant factors in metabolic syndrome. The interplay between ghrelin and leptin further complicates weight management, as these hormones work in opposition to regulate energy homeostasis.

The interaction between these hormones illustrates the complex physiological responses involved in metabolic syndrome. Disruption in the balance of leptin, cortisol, and ghrelin can create a cycle of cravings, stress, and weight gain that perpetuates metabolic dysfunction. Addressing hormonal imbalances through lifestyle modifications, including diet and exercise, is essential for reversing the effects of metabolic syndrome.

In conclusion, understanding the roles of leptin, cortisol, and ghrelin is vital for anyone looking to comprehend metabolic syndrome. By recognising how these hormones influence appetite, stress response, and fat distribution, individuals can better equip themselves to manage their health. Strategies aimed at restoring hormonal balance can lead to significant improvements in metabolic health and overall well-being.

Sedentary Lifestyle and Poor Diet Patterns

A sedentary lifestyle has become increasingly prevalent in today's society, with many individuals spending hours engaged in activities that require little to no physical movement. This lack of activity can lead to a variety of health issues, including obesity, cardiovascular diseases, and ultimately, metabolic syndrome. The convenience of modern technology often contributes to this trend, as many people opt for sedentary forms of entertainment and work, further exacerbating the problem.

In addition to a sedentary lifestyle, poor dietary patterns play a significant role in the development of metabolic syndrome. Many individuals consume diets high in processed foods, sugars, and unhealthy fats, which can lead to insulin resistance and weight gain. These dietary habits are often influenced by busy lifestyles, where convenience takes precedence over nutritional value, resulting in a reliance on fast food and sugary snacks.

The combination of inactivity and poor nutrition creates a vicious cycle that is difficult to break. Individuals may find themselves trapped in a routine where they feel lethargic due to lack of exercise, leading to further unhealthy eating choices. This cycle not only affects physical health but also has detrimental effects on mental well-being, causing feelings of stress and depression that can further perpetuate poor lifestyle choices.

Raising awareness about the impacts of a sedentary lifestyle and poor diet is crucial for preventing metabolic syndrome. Educational initiatives can help individuals understand the importance of incorporating physical activity and making healthier food choices into their daily routines. Simple changes, such as taking regular breaks from sitting or opting for a nutritious meal instead of fast food, can significantly improve health outcomes.

Ultimately, addressing the issues of sedentary behaviour and unhealthy eating is vital for breaking the cycle of metabolic syndrome. By promoting a more active lifestyle and encouraging better dietary habits, individuals can take proactive steps towards preventing this condition. It is essential for everyone to recognise the importance of these factors in maintaining their health and well-being, fostering a culture of wellness in our communities.

3

Chapter 3: Risk Factors and Early Warning Signs

Who's Most at Risk?

Metabolic syndrome is a complex condition that affects millions globally, but certain groups are more susceptible than others. Individuals with a family history of diabetes or cardiovascular disease are at a heightened risk. Genetic predispositions can significantly influence how one's body processes fats and sugars, leading to an increased likelihood of developing these health issues. Understanding these familial patterns can be crucial for preventative measures.

Age is another significant factor in determining risk for metabolic syndrome. As people get older, the likelihood of developing conditions such as obesity, hypertension, and insulin resistance rises. The ageing process can lead to metabolic changes that make it more challenging to maintain a healthy weight and manage blood pressure levels. Therefore, older adults should be particularly vigilant about their health and lifestyle choices.

Lifestyle choices play a critical role in the development of metabolic syndrome. Sedentary behaviour, poor diet, and excessive alcohol consumption can all contribute to the onset of this condition. Individuals who lead inactive lifestyles are more likely to experience weight gain and related health problems. Thus, promoting physical activity and healthy eating habits is essential for everyone, especially those in higher-risk categories.

Gender can also influence the susceptibility to metabolic syndrome. Research indicates that men are generally at a higher risk compared to women, particularly in terms of abdominal obesity. However, post-menopausal women may experience an increased risk due to hormonal changes that affect metabolism. Recognising these differences can lead to more tailored prevention strategies for each gender.

Lastly, certain ethnic groups are more prone to metabolic syndrome, with higher prevalence rates observed in Hispanic, African American, and Native American populations. Socioeconomic factors often intersect with these ethnic disparities, influencing access to healthcare, education, and healthy food options. Addressing these inequalities is vital for effective prevention and management of metabolic syndrome across diverse communities.

Pre-diabetes, PCOS, and Fatty Liver

Pre-diabetes, polycystic ovary syndrome (PCOS), and fatty liver are three interconnected health issues that are increasingly prevalent in today's society. Each condition can significantly impact an individual's metabolic health and overall well-being. Pre-diabetes is often a precursor to type 2 diabetes, characterised by elevated blood glucose levels that are not yet high enough for a diabetes diagnosis. This condition is a warning sign that should not be ignored, as it can lead to more severe metabolic complications if left unaddressed.

PCOS is a hormonal disorder that affects women of reproductive age and is closely linked to insulin resistance, a common feature of metabolic syndrome. Women with PCOS may experience irregular menstrual cycles, weight gain, and fertility issues, all stemming from metabolic dysfunction. The presence of insulin resistance in these individuals not only exacerbates the symptoms of PCOS but also increases the risk of developing pre-diabetes and diabetes later in life.

Fatty liver disease, particularly non-alcoholic fatty liver disease (NAFLD), is another condition that often coexists with pre-diabetes and PCOS. This condition is characterised by the accumulation of fat in liver cells, which can lead to liver inflammation and damage. Insulin resistance is a major contributor to fatty liver, making it crucial for individuals with both pre-diabetes and PCOS to be aware of their liver health and take proactive steps to manage their condition.

The interplay between these three conditions highlights the importance of a holistic approach to health. Lifestyle modifications, such as a balanced diet rich in whole foods, regular physical activity, and weight management, can significantly improve insulin sensitivity and reduce the risk of complications associated with pre-diabetes, PCOS, and fatty liver. Early intervention is vital, as addressing these metabolic issues can lead to a better quality of life and long-term health outcomes.

In conclusion, understanding the connection between pre-diabetes, PCOS, and fatty liver is essential for effective management and prevention strategies. Individuals affected by these conditions should work closely with healthcare professionals to develop personalised plans that address their unique needs. By taking control of their metabolic health, individuals can reduce the risk of developing more severe complications and improve their overall well-being.

Fatty Liver Disease as a Red Flag

Fatty liver disease has emerged as a significant health concern, often acting as a red flag for individuals at risk of developing more severe metabolic conditions. This condition is characterised by an excess accumulation of fat in liver cells, which can lead to inflammation and scarring over time. As the prevalence of obesity and sedentary lifestyles continues to rise, fatty liver disease serves as a crucial indicator of metabolic syndrome, highlighting the need for increased awareness and proactive health management.

The relationship between fatty liver disease and metabolic syndrome is well-established. Individuals with fatty liver disease often exhibit other components of metabolic syndrome, including hypertension, high blood sugar, and dyslipidaemia. The presence of fatty liver can signal underlying insulin resistance, which is a common thread linking these metabolic disorders. Recognising fatty liver disease as a warning sign can empower individuals to make lifestyle changes that may prevent the progression to more serious health issues, such as type 2 diabetes and cardiovascular disease.

Detection of fatty liver disease typically involves imaging tests and blood work. Symptoms may be absent in the early stages, making regular check-ups essential for early diagnosis. Healthcare providers can use these findings to recommend lifestyle interventions, such as improved diet and increased physical activity. By addressing fatty liver disease early, individuals can significantly reduce their risk of developing further complications associated with metabolic syndrome.

Moreover, the educational aspect of fatty liver disease cannot be overlooked. Raising awareness about its implications and the importance of a healthy lifestyle can lead to better outcomes. Community programmes, healthcare campaigns, and educational resources can play pivotal roles in informing the public about the risks associated with fatty liver disease and metabolic syndrome. A well-informed population is better equipped to manage their health and make informed decisions about their lifestyle choices.

In conclusion, fatty liver disease is not merely a benign condition but a crucial red flag in the context of metabolic syndrome. Understanding its implications can lead to timely interventions that may alter the course of an individual's health trajectory. By recognising the signs and symptoms, seeking appropriate medical advice, and committing to healthier lifestyle choices, individuals can combat the rising tide of metabolic syndrome and its associated risks.

Waist-to-Hip Ratio and Body Fat Distribution

The waist-to-hip ratio (WHR) is a crucial measurement that helps assess body fat distribution and potential health risks associated with metabolic syndrome. By comparing the circumference of the waist to that of the hips, individuals can gain insights into their body fat levels. This ratio is particularly significant because it highlights how fat is distributed in the body, which can be more telling than weight alone in terms of health outcomes.

Research indicates that a higher waist-to-hip ratio is linked to an increased risk of cardiovascular diseases, type 2 diabetes, and other metabolic disorders. This is primarily due to the fact that abdominal fat, which contributes to a larger waist circumference, is more metabolically active and poses greater health risks than fat located in the hips or thighs. Understanding this relationship reinforces the importance of monitoring body fat distribution rather than solely focusing on overall weight.

Moreover, the waist-to-hip ratio can serve as a practical tool for individuals to assess their own health without the need for complex equipment. By measuring their waist and hip circumferences with a simple tape measure, anyone can calculate their WHR and identify whether they fall within the recommended ranges. Health professionals often use these measurements as part of routine assessments in various clinical settings to encourage lifestyle modifications when necessary.

It is essential to note that the recommended waist-to-hip ratio varies among different populations and may be influenced by factors such as age, ethnicity, and gender. For instance, a WHR of 0.85 or less is typically considered healthy for women, while a ratio of 0.90 or less is deemed acceptable for men. These thresholds are vital for identifying individuals at higher risk of developing metabolic syndrome and associated health complications.

In conclusion, the waist-to-hip ratio is a significant indicator of body fat distribution and an essential tool in understanding metabolic syndrome. By acknowledging the importance of WHR alongside other measurements, individuals can take proactive steps towards improving their health. Regular monitoring can empower people to make informed choices regarding their lifestyle and dietary habits, ultimately helping to reduce the risk of serious health conditions.

Blood Tests and What They Mean (Fasting glucose, HbA1c, TG, HDL, etc.)

Blood tests are essential in assessing an individual's health, especially concerning metabolic syndrome. Among the various tests, fasting glucose levels are crucial in monitoring blood sugar control. A fasting glucose test measures the sugar level in the blood after an overnight fast, providing insight into how well the body manages glucose. Elevated levels may indicate insulin resistance, which is a key component of metabolic syndrome.

Another important metric is HbA1c, which reflects average blood glucose levels over the past two to three months. This test is particularly useful for diagnosing diabetes and prediabetes, as it showcases how the body has been handling sugar over time. An HbA1c level of 5.7% to 6.4% suggests prediabetes, while a level of 6.5% or higher indicates diabetes, making it a vital tool in understanding one's risk for metabolic disorders.

Triglycerides (TG) are another critical component measured in blood tests. High levels of triglycerides can contribute to the hardening of arteries, increasing the risk of heart disease. A triglyceride level above 150 mg/dL is considered high, and managing this level is essential for individuals at risk of metabolic syndrome. Lifestyle modifications, such as improved diet and increased physical activity, can help lower triglyceride levels.

High-density lipoprotein (HDL) cholesterol, often referred to as 'good' cholesterol, is also a significant marker. Higher levels of HDL can reduce the risk of heart disease, whereas low levels are a concern. An HDL level of less than 40 mg/dL in men and less than 50 mg/dL in women is considered low and may indicate an increased risk of cardiovascular complications. Thus, monitoring HDL levels is crucial for overall metabolic health.

Understanding these blood test results can empower individuals to take charge of their health. Regular testing and awareness of fasting glucose, HbA1c, triglycerides, and HDL levels can guide lifestyle choices and medical interventions. By interpreting these markers correctly, one can better manage metabolic syndrome and improve overall well-being.

4

Chapter 4: Nutrition for Reversing Metabolic Syndrome

The Role of Carbohydrates: Quality over Quantity

Carbohydrates have long been a focal point in discussions about nutrition, particularly concerning their impact on metabolic health. While many people focus on the quantity of carbohydrates consumed, it is essential to consider the quality of these carbohydrates as well. High-quality carbohydrates, such as whole grains, fruits, and vegetables, provide not only energy but also vital nutrients and fibre that are beneficial for overall health. In contrast, low-quality carbohydrates, often found in processed foods, can lead to spikes in blood sugar and ultimately contribute to metabolic syndrome.

The body processes different types of carbohydrates in various ways, and understanding this can aid in making healthier choices. Complex carbohydrates, which are digested more slowly, help maintain stable blood glucose levels, making them a better choice for those concerned about metabolic syndrome. On the other hand, simple carbohydrates, particularly those from refined sources, can disrupt metabolic balance, leading to insulin resistance. By prioritising complex carbohydrates, individuals can enhance their metabolic health significantly.

Moreover, the glycaemic index (GI) is a useful tool for assessing carbohydrate quality. Foods with a low GI are digested slowly and provide a steady release of glucose into the bloodstream, which is particularly advantageous for those managing metabolic syndrome. Incorporating low-GI foods such as legumes, sweet potatoes, and most fruits into one's diet can help mitigate the risks associated with high insulin levels and inflammation, both of which are linked to metabolic disorders.

In addition to focusing on the type of carbohydrates consumed, it is crucial to consider portion sizes and overall dietary balance. Even healthy carbohydrates can contribute to weight gain if consumed in excessive amounts. A well-rounded diet should include a variety of nutrients from all food groups, ensuring that carbohydrates complement proteins and fats rather than dominate the meal. This balance supports metabolic health and prevents the adverse effects associated with carbohydrate overconsumption.

Ultimately, embracing the idea of quality over quantity when it comes to carbohydrates can lead to improved metabolic health and overall well-being. By making informed choices about the types of carbohydrates consumed, individuals can better manage their weight, enhance their energy levels, and reduce the risk of developing serious health issues associated with metabolic syndrome. Understanding the role of carbohydrates in our diet is a vital step towards achieving optimal health and longevity.

Low-Glycemic and Anti-Inflammatory Eating

Low-glycemic and anti-inflammatory eating is an essential approach for managing metabolic syndrome. This dietary strategy focuses on foods that have a minimal impact on blood sugar levels, helping to stabilise insulin and glucose responses. By incorporating whole foods such as vegetables, lean proteins, and healthy fats, individuals can significantly improve their metabolic health and reduce the risk of chronic diseases associated with metabolic syndrome.

The low-glycemic index (GI) concept revolves around selecting carbohydrates that are digested and absorbed slowly. These foods cause a gradual rise in blood sugar levels, preventing spikes that can lead to inflammation and insulin resistance. Examples include whole grains, legumes, and most fruits and vegetables, which provide essential nutrients while maintaining stable energy levels.

In addition to focusing on low-GI foods, it is crucial to include anti-inflammatory ingredients in one's diet. Foods rich in antioxidants, such as berries, leafy greens, and nuts, can help reduce inflammation within the body. Omega-3 fatty acids, found in fish and flaxseeds, also play a significant role in combating inflammation and promoting heart health, which is particularly important for those dealing with metabolic syndrome.

Hydration is another key aspect of a low-glycemic and anti-inflammatory diet. Drinking plenty of water and herbal teas can aid in maintaining proper metabolic function and reducing inflammation. Avoiding sugary drinks and excessive caffeine is advisable, as these can contribute to blood sugar spikes and inflammatory responses.

To conclude, adopting a low-glycemic and anti-inflammatory eating pattern can have profound effects on individuals with metabolic syndrome. By making informed food choices and prioritising nutrient-dense options, it is possible to enhance overall health, manage weight, and significantly lower the risk of associated complications. This dietary approach not only benefits metabolic syndrome but contributes to a healthier lifestyle overall.

Protein and Healthy Fats for Satiety and Insulin Balance

Protein and healthy fats play a crucial role in promoting satiety and maintaining insulin balance, which are essential for overall metabolic health. When we consume meals rich in protein, our bodies experience a greater feeling of fullness compared to those high in carbohydrates or sugars. This is largely due to the way protein influences hormones that regulate appetite, such as ghrelin and peptide YY. By including adequate protein in our diets, we can help to curb hunger and reduce the likelihood of overeating, which is particularly beneficial for individuals managing metabolic syndrome.

In addition to protein, healthy fats are instrumental in enhancing satiety.

Unlike refined carbohydrates, which can lead to quick spikes and subsequent drops in blood sugar levels, healthy fats provide a more stable source of energy. Foods such as avocados, nuts, and olive oil not only satisfy hunger but also contribute to the absorption of fat-soluble vitamins. The combination of protein and healthy fats in meals can lead to a more balanced blood sugar response, reducing the risk of insulin resistance associated with metabolic syndrome.

Another vital aspect of incorporating protein and healthy fats into our diets is their impact on our overall dietary patterns. Emphasising these macronutrients can naturally lead to a reduction in the intake of processed foods high in sugars and unhealthy fats. This shift towards whole, nutrient-dense foods can foster better dietary habits and support long-term health. Moreover, it encourages mindful eating practices, which are essential for maintaining a healthy weight and managing metabolic syndrome effectively.

It is also important to consider the quality of the protein and fats we choose. Opting for lean sources of protein, such as fish, chicken, and legumes, alongside unsaturated fats, can optimise health benefits. Additionally, avoiding trans fats and limiting saturated fats can further enhance metabolic health. By prioritising high-quality food sources, individuals can improve their insulin sensitivity and overall well-being, making it easier to manage metabolic syndrome.

In conclusion, incorporating protein and healthy fats into our diets is a strategic approach to achieving satiety and maintaining insulin balance. These macronutrients not only help control appetite but also foster healthier eating behaviours and improve metabolic outcomes. Understanding the roles of protein and fats can empower individuals to make informed dietary choices that support their health, particularly for those facing the challenges of metabolic syndrome.

Sample Meal Plans and Grocery List

When it comes to managing metabolic syndrome, having a structured meal plan can significantly aid in achieving better health outcomes. A well-balanced diet that is rich in whole foods while being low in processed items can help individuals control their weight, blood sugar levels, and cholesterol. Sample meal plans can serve as a practical guide, providing a variety of options that cater to different tastes and nutritional needs. The inclusion of fresh fruits, vegetables, whole grains, and lean proteins is paramount in these plans to ensure all essential nutrients are consumed daily.

For a typical day's meal plan, breakfast might consist of oatmeal topped with berries and a sprinkle of nuts, which provides a hearty start to the day. Lunch could feature a quinoa salad with mixed greens, cherry tomatoes, and grilled chicken, dressed lightly with olive oil and lemon juice. Dinner may include baked salmon with steamed broccoli and brown rice, ensuring a balance of omega-3 fatty acids and fibre. Healthy snacks such as carrot sticks with hummus or a piece of fruit can help maintain energy levels between meals, preventing unhealthy cravings.

In addition to meal planning, a well-thought-out grocery list is crucial for successful implementation. A grocery list should focus on whole foods such as fresh produce, whole grains like brown rice and quinoa, lean proteins such as chicken, fish, and legumes, as well as healthy fats found in nuts, seeds, and avocados. By planning ahead, individuals can avoid impulse purchases of processed and unhealthy foods that may derail their progress in managing metabolic syndrome.

It is also beneficial to keep in mind portion control when preparing meals. Understanding serving sizes can help prevent overeating, which is essential for those with metabolic syndrome. Including a variety of colours on the plate not only makes meals visually appealing but also ensures a range of nutrients. It is recommended to drink plenty of water throughout the day, as staying hydrated plays a vital role in overall health and can assist in weight management.

Ultimately, the key to success in managing metabolic syndrome lies in consistency and commitment to a healthier lifestyle. By adhering to structured meal plans and maintaining a comprehensive grocery list, individuals can take substantial steps towards improving their health. Regularly revisiting and adjusting meal plans to suit personal preferences and seasonal availability can keep the diet interesting and enjoyable, making it easier to adhere to in the long run.

Addressing Sugar Addiction and Emotional Eating

Sugar addiction and emotional eating are significant factors contributing to metabolic syndrome. Individuals often turn to sugary foods as a means of coping with stress or negative emotions, leading to a cycle of dependence that can be difficult to break. Understanding this connection is crucial in addressing the root causes of metabolic syndrome, as these behaviours not only affect physical health but also emotional well-being.

Recognising triggers for sugar cravings is the first step in overcoming addiction. Common triggers may include stress, boredom, or social situations that encourage unhealthy eating habits. By identifying these triggers, individuals can develop healthier coping mechanisms, such as engaging in physical activity or practising mindfulness, which can help mitigate the urge to consume sugary foods.

Another essential aspect of addressing sugar addiction is educating oneself on nutrition and the impact of sugar on the body. Many people are unaware of how quickly sugar can affect mood and energy levels, leading to a cycle of highs and lows. A better understanding of nutritional labels and the hidden sugars in processed foods can empower individuals to make informed choices, ultimately leading to better health outcomes.

Support systems play a vital role in combating emotional eating and sugar addiction. Surrounding oneself with friends, family, or support groups can provide encouragement and accountability. Sharing experiences with others who understand the challenges can create a sense of community, making it easier to navigate the journey toward healthier eating habits.

Finally, seeking professional help may be necessary for those struggling with severe sugar addiction or emotional eating. Therapists and nutritionists can offer tailored guidance and strategies to help individuals develop a healthier relationship with food. By addressing both psychological and nutritional aspects, individuals can break free from the grips of sugar addiction and improve their overall metabolic health.

5

Chapter 5: Intermittent Fasting and Time-Restricted Eating

How It Works and Why It Helps

Metabolic syndrome is a complex cluster of conditions that increase the risk of heart disease, stroke, and diabetes. Understanding how it works is crucial for managing health effectively. The syndrome typically involves a combination of increased blood pressure, high blood sugar levels, excess body fat around the waist, and abnormal cholesterol levels. Each of these factors is interlinked, creating a vicious cycle that exacerbates health risks. By grasping the underlying mechanisms, individuals can take proactive steps towards prevention and management.

The way metabolic syndrome operates is largely influenced by lifestyle choices and genetic predispositions. Poor diet, lack of physical activity, and obesity are contributing factors that can trigger this syndrome. When the body accumulates excess fat, particularly visceral fat around the abdomen, it leads to insulin resistance. This means that the body's cells do not respond effectively to insulin, causing elevated blood sugar levels. Understanding this correlation helps individuals recognise the importance of maintaining a healthy lifestyle to mitigate risks associated with metabolic syndrome.

Addressing metabolic syndrome can significantly enhance overall health and well-being. Interventions such as dietary changes, increased physical activity, and medical management can reverse the effects of the syndrome. For instance, adopting a balanced diet rich in whole foods can improve cholesterol levels and reduce blood pressure. Regular exercise not only aids weight loss but also enhances insulin sensitivity. By implementing these strategies, individuals can improve their metabolic health and reduce the likelihood of developing serious complications.

Furthermore, awareness and education about metabolic syndrome can empower individuals to make informed decisions regarding their health. Regular health check-ups and screenings can help detect early signs of the syndrome, allowing for timely intervention. Support from healthcare professionals, as well as community programmes focused on lifestyle changes, can provide the necessary resources to facilitate these improvements. Understanding the 'why' behind these changes reinforces the importance of taking responsibility for one's health.

In summary, understanding how metabolic syndrome works and why it helps to address it is vital for individuals seeking to improve their health outcomes. The interplay of lifestyle, genetics, and medical intervention plays a critical role in managing this syndrome. By prioritising education and awareness, individuals can take charge of their health, ultimately leading to a healthier and more active life. Embracing these changes not only benefits personal health but also contributes to the wider community's well-being.

Different Methods: 16:8, 5:2, Eat-Stop-Eat

Intermittent fasting has gained significant popularity for its potential health benefits, particularly in relation to metabolic syndrome. Among the various methods available, the 16:8, 5:2, and Eat-Stop-Eat approaches stand out for their simplicity and effectiveness. The 16:8 method involves fasting for 16 hours each day and eating within an 8-hour window, which can easily fit into most lifestyles. This technique encourages individuals to skip breakfast and consume their meals between noon and 8 PM, allowing them to align their eating patterns with their natural circadian rhythms.

The 5:2 method offers a different approach, where individuals consume a normal diet for five days of the week and restrict calorie intake to about 500-600 calories on two non-consecutive days. This method can be particularly appealing for those who struggle with strict daily fasting, as it provides flexibility while still promoting weight loss and improved metabolic health. Research suggests that this approach can help reduce insulin resistance, a key factor in metabolic syndrome, by allowing the body to enter a state of ketosis on fasting days.

Eat-Stop-Eat is another intermittent fasting strategy that involves a 24-hour fast once or twice a week. Participants may choose to fast from dinner one day to dinner the next, or from lunch to lunch. This method can be more challenging due to the length of the fasting period, but it has been associated with significant health benefits, including improved blood sugar control and reduced inflammation. It is essential for individuals considering this method to stay hydrated and to break their fasts with nutritious foods to maximise health benefits.

Each of these methods has its advantages and potential drawbacks, making it crucial for individuals to choose the one that best fits their lifestyle and health goals. Consulting with a healthcare professional can provide guidance tailored to individual needs, especially for those with existing health conditions like metabolic syndrome. Understanding personal responses to fasting can also help in determining which method is more sustainable in the long run.

In conclusion, the 16:8, 5:2, and Eat-Stop-Eat methods of intermittent fasting offer viable options for managing metabolic syndrome. They promote weight loss, improve metabolic health, and can be adapted to suit various lifestyles. As interest in these methods continues to grow, ongoing research will likely provide further insights into their long-term effectiveness and safety for individuals seeking to improve their health through dietary changes.

Who Should and Shouldn't Try It

Metabolic syndrome is a condition that affects a significant number of individuals across diverse demographics. However, not everyone is equally suited to attempt lifestyle changes aimed at reversing or managing this syndrome. Generally, those who are at risk for metabolic syndrome, including individuals with obesity, hypertension, or diabetes, should seriously consider making alterations to their diet and exercise routines. These individuals stand to benefit the most from targeted strategies that can alleviate symptoms and improve overall health outcomes.

On the other hand, certain populations should approach such changes with caution. Individuals with pre-existing health issues, such as heart disease, kidney problems, or severe mental health conditions, may find that aggressive lifestyle changes could pose risks rather than benefits. It is crucial for these individuals to consult with healthcare professionals before embarking on any new health regimen. Personalised advice from medical practitioners ensures that any attempts at lifestyle modification are safe and tailored to individual health needs.

Moreover, those who are already maintaining a healthy lifestyle may not need to engage in drastic changes to their routine. For example, individuals who are physically active, consume a balanced diet, and regularly monitor their health markers may find that they are already managing their metabolic health effectively. Instead of overhauling their lifestyle, they might focus on fine-tuning their existing habits to ensure continued well-being.

In addition to personal health status, age and genetic factors also play a role in determining who should try lifestyle changes related to metabolic syndrome. Older adults may experience more challenges in implementing significant changes due to physical limitations or comorbidities. Similarly, individuals with a family history of metabolic disorders should be particularly vigilant and seek professional guidance to navigate their health journey effectively.

Ultimately, the decision to pursue lifestyle changes in relation to metabolic syndrome should be a well-considered one, taking into account individual health circumstances, genetic predispositions, and existing lifestyle habits.

Engaging with healthcare providers is essential for anyone considering such changes, ensuring that the approach taken is not only beneficial but also safe for their unique situation.

Common Pitfalls and How to Start Safely

Metabolic syndrome is a complex condition that can lead to serious health issues if not managed properly. One of the most common pitfalls individuals face is the misunderstanding of what constitutes a healthy lifestyle. Many people believe that simply losing weight or engaging in sporadic exercise is sufficient to combat the effects of metabolic syndrome. However, it is crucial to adopt a holistic approach that includes balanced nutrition, regular physical activity, and consistent monitoring of health metrics.

Another significant pitfall is the tendency to rely on quick fixes or fad diets. These approaches often promise rapid results but can lead to nutritional deficiencies and unsustainable habits. Individuals are encouraged to seek guidance from healthcare professionals who can provide personalised plans that focus on gradual, sustainable changes rather than drastic measures. This ensures that the body receives the necessary nutrients while effectively managing weight and health.

A lack of awareness about the importance of stress management can also hinder progress. Chronic stress is known to contribute to metabolic dysfunction, and many individuals underestimate its impact on their overall health. Incorporating stress-reduction techniques such as mindfulness, meditation, or engaging in hobbies can greatly enhance one's ability to manage their condition effectively. A well-rounded approach to health should always consider mental and emotional well-being in tandem with physical health.

Social support is another crucial element that people often overlook. Facing metabolic syndrome can be challenging, and having a support network can make a significant difference. Whether it's friends, family, or support groups, sharing experiences and challenges can provide motivation and accountability. This communal aspect of health management can foster a sense of belonging and encouragement that is vital for long-term success.

Lastly, it's essential to start any health journey with realistic expectations. Many individuals become discouraged when they do not see immediate results, leading to feelings of defeat. Setting achievable goals and celebrating small victories can help maintain motivation. Understanding that managing metabolic syndrome is a lifelong journey rather than a sprint can empower individuals to make lasting changes that promote overall health and well-being.

6

Chapter 6: Exercise and Physical Activity

Benefits for Insulin Sensitivity and Fat Burning

Insulin sensitivity and fat burning are crucial components of metabolic health, particularly for individuals at risk of metabolic syndrome. Improved insulin sensitivity means that the body's cells can effectively utilise insulin, leading to better glucose control and reduced blood sugar levels. This physiological change can significantly decrease the risk of type 2 diabetes, a common consequence of metabolic syndrome. By enhancing insulin sensitivity, individuals can also experience improved energy levels and overall vitality.

Fat burning, on the other hand, is essential for weight management and reducing body fat percentage. When the body becomes more efficient at burning fat, particularly during periods of physical activity, it can lead to a healthier body composition. This process not only helps in shedding excess weight but also contributes to cardiovascular health by lowering the risk of obesity-related diseases. A well-regulated metabolism that prioritises fat burning over carbohydrate storage is beneficial for long-term health.

Incorporating regular physical activity is one of the most effective strategies for improving insulin sensitivity and promoting fat burning. Aerobic exercises, strength training, and high-intensity interval training have been shown to have a profound impact on these metabolic processes. Additionally, dietary choices play a significant role; consuming a balanced diet rich in whole foods, healthy fats, and lean proteins can further enhance these benefits. This holistic approach combines lifestyle changes that support metabolic health.

Another factor to consider is the impact of stress and sleep on insulin sensitivity and fat metabolism. Chronic stress can lead to elevated cortisol levels, which may impair insulin sensitivity and encourage fat storage, particularly in the abdominal area. Likewise, inadequate sleep is associated with hormonal imbalances that can disrupt metabolic processes. Prioritising stress management techniques and ensuring sufficient rest can therefore complement physical and dietary efforts in improving metabolic health.

Ultimately, the benefits of enhanced insulin sensitivity and effective fat burning extend beyond mere weight loss. They contribute to a reduced risk of chronic diseases, improved mental health, and a greater overall quality of life. Understanding these benefits empowers individuals to take proactive steps towards better health outcomes, fostering a sense of agency and motivation in their wellness journeys. As awareness of metabolic syndrome grows, so does the importance of promoting practices that support insulin sensitivity and fat burning in everyday life.

Aerobic vs Resistance Training

Aerobic and resistance training are two vital components of a comprehensive fitness regimen, each offering unique benefits that are especially pertinent for individuals managing metabolic syndrome. Aerobic training, which includes activities such as walking, running, swimming, and cycling, primarily focuses on improving cardiovascular health by increasing the efficiency of the heart and lungs. This type of exercise is essential for burning calories and fat, thereby aiding in weight management, which is crucial for those with metabolic syndrome. Regular aerobic exercise has been shown to enhance insulin sensitivity, lower blood pressure, and reduce the risk of heart disease, making it a foundational element of any health strategy.

In contrast, resistance training involves exercises that build muscle strength, endurance, and mass through the use of weights, resistance bands, or bodyweight exercises. This form of exercise is particularly beneficial for increasing lean muscle tissue, which plays a significant role in enhancing metabolic rate. By incorporating resistance training into a fitness routine, individuals can improve their body composition, increase strength, and support better glucose metabolism. This is crucial for those with metabolic syndrome, as higher muscle mass can lead to improved insulin sensitivity and overall metabolic health.

The combination of aerobic and resistance training is particularly effective for individuals with metabolic syndrome, as it addresses multiple aspects of health. While aerobic exercise helps with fat loss and cardiovascular health, resistance training contributes to muscle gain and metabolic enhancement. Studies have indicated that those who engage in both forms of exercise experience greater health improvements compared to those who focus solely on one. Thus, a balanced approach that includes both aerobic and resistance components is recommended for optimal health outcomes.

It is important to note that the intensity and frequency of both aerobic and resistance training should be tailored to individual capabilities and health status. Beginners may start with moderate-intensity aerobic activities for at least 150 minutes per week, alongside resistance training sessions at least two days a week. As fitness levels improve, individuals can gradually increase the intensity and duration of their workouts. Consulting with a healthcare provider or fitness professional can help in designing a safe and effective programme that meets personal health goals.

In summary, understanding the distinctions and complementary benefits of aerobic and resistance training is essential for anyone looking to improve their health, particularly those affected by metabolic syndrome. By integrating both types of exercise, individuals can achieve better weight management, enhanced metabolic function, and reduced risk of associated health conditions. Emphasising a holistic approach to fitness can lead to substantial improvements in overall well-being and quality of life.

NEAT (Non-Exercise Activity Thermogenesis)

NEAT, or Non-Exercise Activity Thermogenesis, refers to the energy expenditure that occurs during daily activities that are not classified as formal exercise. This includes everything from fidgeting and standing to walking around the house or office. In contrast to structured workouts, NEAT can significantly contribute to overall calorie burn and plays a crucial role in maintaining a healthy weight. Understanding NEAT is essential for those looking to manage their metabolic health effectively.

One of the fascinating aspects of NEAT is how it varies among individuals. Factors such as occupation, lifestyle, and even personality traits can influence the amount of energy expended through non-exercise activities. For instance, a person with a physically demanding job may have a higher NEAT compared to someone who works a sedentary office job. Recognising these differences can help individuals tailor their daily routines to enhance their NEAT and, consequently, their metabolic rate.

Incorporating more NEAT into daily life can be a straightforward yet effective strategy for combating sedentary behaviour. Simple actions like taking the stairs instead of the lift, walking during phone calls, or even doing household chores can significantly increase daily calorie expenditure. These activities may seem minor, but when accumulated over time, they can lead to substantial weight management benefits and contribute to overall metabolic health.

Moreover, research indicates that increasing NEAT can provide additional health benefits beyond weight control. Engaging in more physical movement throughout the day can enhance cardiovascular health, improve mood, and boost energy levels. These benefits underscore the importance of staying active, even in small ways, as part of a comprehensive approach to managing metabolic syndrome and overall health.

In conclusion, NEAT is a vital component of daily energy expenditure that everyone can enhance without engaging in formal exercise. By making small adjustments to daily routines and focusing on increasing non-exercise activities, individuals can improve their metabolic health and overall well-being. Embracing NEAT not only aids in weight management but also enriches the quality of life by promoting an active lifestyle.

Building a Weekly Routine That Works

Establishing a weekly routine can significantly impact your overall health, especially when addressing metabolic syndrome. A well-structured routine not only promotes consistency in healthy habits but also aids in managing stress levels, which is crucial for maintaining metabolic balance. Begin by identifying your goals and the specific changes you wish to incorporate into your lifestyle. This foundation will guide you in creating a routine that aligns with your individual needs and capabilities.

Incorporate regular physical activity into your weekly schedule, as it is a key component in managing metabolic syndrome. Aim for at least 150 minutes of moderate aerobic exercise or 75 minutes of vigorous activity each week. This can be broken down into manageable segments, such as 30 minutes a day, five days a week. Engaging in activities that you enjoy can make this routine more sustainable, turning exercise into a rewarding part of your daily life rather than a chore.

Nutrition also plays a vital role in your weekly routine. Plan your meals ahead of time to ensure that you are consuming a balanced diet rich in whole foods, fruits, vegetables, lean proteins, and healthy fats. Preparing meals in advance can help you avoid unhealthy food choices during busy periods. Consider setting aside time each week for grocery shopping and meal prep, which will facilitate healthier eating habits and support your metabolic health.

Mindfulness and stress management techniques should not be overlooked when building your routine. Incorporating practices such as meditation, yoga, or even simple breathing exercises can greatly enhance your mental well-being and help you manage stress effectively. Allocate time each week for these activities, ensuring that you have a dedicated space and time for relaxation and reflection amidst your busy schedule.

Finally, remember to be flexible with your routine. Life can be unpredictable, and it is essential to adapt your plans as necessary. Regularly review and adjust your routine to ensure it remains effective and enjoyable. This flexibility will not only help you stay committed but will also allow you to make long-term changes that contribute positively to managing metabolic syndrome and enhancing your overall health.

Managing Exercise in People with Obesity or Joint Pain

Managing exercise in individuals with obesity or joint pain requires a thoughtful approach that prioritises safety and effectiveness. It is essential to recognise that traditional exercise routines may not be suitable for everyone, particularly those who experience discomfort or limitations due to their weight or underlying joint conditions. Therefore, a tailored programme that considers individual capabilities and preferences is vital for promoting adherence and ensuring long-term success.

Low-impact activities such as swimming, cycling, and walking are often recommended for those managing obesity or joint pain. These forms of exercise help reduce stress on the joints while still providing cardiovascular benefits. Gradually increasing the duration and intensity of these activities can help individuals build strength and endurance without exacerbating their pain or discomfort.

Incorporating flexibility and strength training into the exercise regimen is also crucial. Gentle stretching can enhance mobility and reduce stiffness, while strength training aids in building muscle and supporting joint stability. Resistance exercises using light weights or resistance bands can be particularly beneficial, as they allow individuals to develop strength at their own pace and comfort level.

It is equally important to encourage individuals to listen to their bodies and adjust their exercise routines accordingly. Pain should not be ignored, and modifications should be made to avoid further injury. Consulting with healthcare professionals such as physiotherapists or personal trainers who specialise in working with individuals with obesity or joint pain can provide valuable guidance and support.

Finally, creating a supportive environment that fosters motivation and accountability can significantly enhance exercise adherence. Group classes, community support groups, or online forums can provide encouragement and camaraderie, making the exercise journey more enjoyable. By managing exercise effectively, individuals with obesity or joint pain can improve their overall health, enhance their quality of life, and reduce the risks associated with metabolic syndrome.

7

Chapter 7: Stress, Sleep, and Hormonal Balance

The Cortisol Connection

Cortisol, often referred to as the stress hormone, plays a crucial role in the body's response to stress. It is produced by the adrenal glands and is essential for various functions, including regulating metabolism, reducing inflammation, and controlling the sleep-wake cycle. However, chronic stress can lead to prolonged elevated levels of cortisol, which can have detrimental effects on health, particularly in the context of metabolic syndrome. Understanding the relationship between cortisol and metabolic syndrome is essential for managing and preventing this condition.

Research indicates that high cortisol levels can lead to increased appetite and cravings for unhealthy foods, particularly those high in sugar and fat. This can result in weight gain, particularly around the abdomen, which is a significant risk factor for developing metabolic syndrome. Furthermore, elevated cortisol may also promote insulin resistance, making it more challenging for the body to regulate blood sugar levels effectively. This interplay between cortisol and insulin is vital in understanding how stress can contribute to metabolic disorders.

Additionally, cortisol can influence other hormones and neurotransmitters that are involved in mood and behaviour. Chronic high levels of cortisol are associated with anxiety and depression, which can further perpetuate unhealthy eating habits and sedentary lifestyles. This cycle creates a feedback loop that exacerbates the risk of metabolic syndrome. Therefore, addressing stress and cortisol levels is not only important for mental health but also crucial for physical health.

Strategies to manage cortisol levels include regular physical activity, mindfulness practices, and adequate sleep. Exercise has been shown to reduce cortisol levels and improve overall well-being. Mindfulness and relaxation techniques can also be effective in mitigating stress responses, thereby helping to lower cortisol production. Furthermore, ensuring consistent and restorative sleep patterns plays a significant role in maintaining healthy cortisol levels and preventing metabolic syndrome.

In conclusion, the connection between cortisol and metabolic syndrome is multifaceted and significant. By understanding this relationship, individuals can take proactive steps to manage stress and maintain healthier cortisol levels, ultimately reducing their risk of metabolic syndrome. Emphasising the importance of a holistic approach that includes lifestyle modifications will empower individuals to take charge of their health and well-being, leading to better outcomes in the long run.

How Sleep Affects Weight and Metabolism

Sleep plays a crucial role in regulating weight and metabolism, influencing various hormonal functions that govern appetite and energy expenditure. Insufficient sleep can lead to hormonal imbalances, particularly in leptin and ghrelin, which control hunger signals. When we do not get enough quality sleep, our bodies may produce more ghrelin, the hormone that stimulates appetite, while reducing leptin, the hormone that signals fullness. This imbalance can lead to increased cravings and overeating, contributing to weight gain over time.

Moreover, poor sleep quality can directly affect our metabolism. Lack of sleep is linked to reduced insulin sensitivity, which means the body becomes less effective at processing glucose. This can increase the risk of developing metabolic syndrome, a cluster of conditions that includes increased blood pressure, high blood sugar levels, excess body fat around the waist, and abnormal cholesterol levels. When metabolism is sluggish, it becomes more difficult to maintain a healthy weight, leading to further complications.

The impact of sleep on physical activity is also significant. Individuals who are sleep-deprived often experience fatigue, making them less likely to engage in regular exercise. This reduction in physical activity not only hinders weight loss efforts but can also contribute to muscle loss, which is vital for maintaining a healthy metabolic rate. A well-rested body is more energised and better equipped to perform physical activities, thereby promoting a more efficient metabolism.

In addition to these physiological effects, sleep quality is influenced by lifestyle choices that can also affect weight management. Factors such as stress, diet, and screen time before bed can disrupt sleep patterns. Addressing these lifestyle factors can lead to improved sleep quality, which in turn supports a healthier metabolism and weight. Prioritising good sleep hygiene is essential to mitigate the effects of metabolic syndrome and to foster overall well-being.

Ultimately, understanding the relationship between sleep, weight, and metabolism is vital for anyone looking to improve their health. By recognising the importance of quality sleep, individuals can make informed choices that support not only weight management but also metabolic health. Emphasising good sleep practices can lead to a more balanced hormonal environment, improved energy levels, and a healthier body composition, providing a solid foundation for overall health and longevity.

Tools for Better Sleep Hygiene

Achieving better sleep hygiene is essential for maintaining overall health and can play a crucial role in managing metabolic syndrome. The tools for improving sleep hygiene include creating a consistent sleep schedule, making your sleeping environment conducive to rest, and practising relaxation techniques. A regular sleep routine helps regulate the body's internal clock, making it easier to fall asleep and wake up, which can positively influence metabolic health.

Stress Management: Mindfulness, CBT, Breathing Techniques

Stress management is a crucial aspect of maintaining overall health, particularly for individuals dealing with metabolic syndrome. Mindfulness is a powerful technique that encourages individuals to focus on the present moment, helping to reduce anxiety and promote a sense of calm. By practising mindfulness, one can develop greater awareness of thoughts and feelings, which allows for better emotional regulation and resilience against stressors.

Cognitive Behavioural Therapy (CBT) is another effective tool for managing stress. This therapeutic approach focuses on identifying and challenging negative thought patterns that contribute to stress. By reframing these thoughts, individuals can change their emotional responses and behaviours, leading to a more balanced and less stressful life. CBT equips individuals with practical strategies to cope with everyday challenges, making it a valuable resource in stress management.

Breathing techniques also play a significant role in alleviating stress. Simple exercises, such as deep breathing or the 4-7-8 technique, can activate the body's relaxation response, reducing tension and promoting a sense of peace. Incorporating these techniques into daily routines can enhance one's ability to cope with stress and improve overall mental clarity, which is particularly beneficial for those managing metabolic syndrome.

Combining mindfulness, CBT, and breathing techniques creates a comprehensive approach to stress management. Each method complements the other, offering a holistic strategy that addresses both the mind and body. By integrating these practices, individuals can build resilience, enhance their mental well-being, and ultimately support their physical health in the face of metabolic syndrome.

Incorporating these stress management techniques into daily life can lead to significant improvements in overall health. Emphasising the importance of mental well-being is essential for those dealing with metabolic syndrome, as stress can exacerbate physical symptoms. By prioritising mindfulness, CBT, and effective breathing techniques, individuals can take proactive steps towards a healthier and more balanced life.

8

Chapter 8: The Role of Medications and Supplements

Metformin, GLP-1 Agonists (e.g., Ozempic, Semaglutide)

Metformin and GLP-1 agonists, such as Ozempic and Semaglutide, play pivotal roles in the management of metabolic syndrome, particularly in patients with type 2 diabetes. Metformin, a first-line medication, primarily works by improving insulin sensitivity and reducing hepatic glucose production. This dual action not only aids in blood sugar control but also contributes to weight management, making it a cornerstone in treating individuals with metabolic disorders.

GLP-1 agonists, on the other hand, are a newer class of medications that mimic the incretin hormone, which enhances insulin secretion in response to food intake. Ozempic and Semaglutide have gained popularity due to their efficacy in promoting weight loss and improving glycaemic control. These medications not only help in managing blood sugar levels but also have cardiovascular benefits, reducing the risk of heart disease in patients with metabolic syndrome.

The combination of Metformin and GLP-1 agonists offers a comprehensive approach to treating metabolic syndrome. While Metformin addresses insulin resistance, GLP-1 agonists help regulate appetite and promote satiety. This synergy can lead to significant improvements in overall health, as patients often experience weight loss, better blood sugar control, and enhanced quality of life.

It is essential for healthcare providers to consider individual patient needs when prescribing these medications. Factors such as the patient's weight, glucose levels, and cardiovascular risk should guide the treatment plan. Additionally, monitoring for potential side effects, such as gastrointestinal issues with Metformin or nausea with GLP-1 agonists, is crucial to ensure patient compliance and effectiveness of the therapy.

In conclusion, Metformin and GLP-1 agonists like Ozempic and Semaglutide represent significant advancements in the treatment of metabolic syndrome. Their unique mechanisms of action not only address the critical components of this syndrome but also promote a healthier lifestyle through weight management and improved metabolic health. As research continues to evolve, these medications will undoubtedly play an integral role in combating the global epidemic of metabolic syndrome.

Supplements: Omega-3, Berberine, Magnesium, Vitamin D

Supplements play a significant role in managing metabolic syndrome, with several key nutrients showing promising benefits. Omega-3 fatty acids are well-known for their anti-inflammatory properties and their ability to improve cardiovascular health. Studies have indicated that these fats can help lower triglyceride levels and may even assist in reducing the risk of heart disease, a major concern for those with metabolic syndrome. Incorporating omega-3s through diet or supplementation can be an effective strategy for promoting overall health.

Another supplement of interest is berberine, a compound found in various plants that has gained attention for its ability to help regulate blood sugar levels. Research suggests that berberine can enhance insulin sensitivity and improve lipid profiles, making it a valuable addition for individuals struggling with metabolic syndrome. Its ability to support weight management through metabolic pathways further underscores its potential as a therapeutic agent.

Magnesium is another crucial mineral that often goes overlooked in discussions about metabolic health. It plays a vital role in numerous biochemical reactions in the body, including those involved in glucose metabolism and blood pressure regulation. Adequate magnesium intake has been associated with a lower risk of type 2 diabetes and cardiovascular disease, making it an essential component of a holistic approach to managing metabolic syndrome.

Vitamin D, often referred to as the sunshine vitamin, also merits attention in the context of metabolic syndrome. Research has linked low levels of vitamin D to increased risks of obesity, insulin resistance, and cardiovascular disorders. Supplementing with vitamin D may not only help in maintaining bone health but could also play a role in improving metabolic outcomes, particularly in individuals with low serum levels of this important nutrient.

In conclusion, the integration of supplements such as omega-3, berberine, magnesium, and vitamin D can provide a multifaceted approach to managing metabolic syndrome. Each of these supplements offers unique benefits that can contribute to improved metabolic health. However, it is essential to consult with healthcare professionals before starting any supplementation regimen to ensure safety and appropriateness for individual health needs.

Risks of Relying Solely on Pills

Relying solely on pills to manage metabolic syndrome can pose significant risks. Many individuals may be tempted to believe that medication alone will solve their health issues without addressing underlying lifestyle factors. This mindset can lead to neglecting essential components such as diet, exercise, and stress management, which are critical for long-term health improvement. As a result, the reliance on pharmaceutical solutions may become a double-edged sword, offering short-term relief while potentially exacerbating the condition over time.

One of the most pressing concerns is the side effects associated with long-term use of medication. Many prescription drugs can lead to unwanted health complications, including weight gain, cardiovascular issues, and even dependency. Moreover, individuals might find themselves in a cycle of increasing dosages as their bodies adapt to the medication, which can further complicate their health status. This can create a false sense of security, as the underlying metabolic issues remain unaddressed, ultimately leading to more severe health consequences.

In addition, the financial burden of relying on pills should not be underestimated. Prescription medications can be costly, and without a comprehensive lifestyle approach to managing metabolic syndrome, individuals may find themselves spending significant amounts of money on treatments that only provide symptomatic relief. This can divert funds away from healthier choices, such as nutritious foods and fitness programs, which are crucial for managing the syndrome effectively.

Furthermore, the psychological impact of relying solely on medication can be detrimental. Individuals may develop a dependency on these drugs, leading to feelings of helplessness regarding their health. This mental state can hinder motivation to adopt healthier lifestyle changes, as the focus shifts solely to medication as a solution. Consequently, the individual may become trapped in a cycle of reliance, further impacting their overall well-being and quality of life.

Ultimately, a holistic approach that combines medication with lifestyle changes is essential for effectively managing metabolic syndrome. This means recognising the limitations of pills and understanding that they should be part of a broader strategy that includes dietary adjustments, physical activity, and psychological support. By doing so, individuals can reclaim control over their health and significantly reduce the risks associated with relying solely on pharmaceutical interventions.

Integrative Approaches: When Medicine and Lifestyle Meet

Integrative approaches to health focus on the synergy between traditional medicine and lifestyle changes in managing metabolic syndrome. This condition, characterised by a cluster of risk factors including obesity, hypertension, and insulin resistance, often requires more than just medication for effective management. By combining medical treatments with lifestyle modifications, patients can achieve better overall health outcomes and reduce their risk of serious complications.

One key aspect of integrative approaches is the emphasis on diet. Nutritional interventions, such as adopting a Mediterranean or a low-carbohydrate diet, have shown promise in improving metabolic health. These dietary strategies not only help with weight management but also enhance insulin sensitivity, making them vital components of a comprehensive treatment plan.

Physical activity is another cornerstone of integrative health. Regular exercise contributes to weight loss, lowers blood pressure, and improves cardiovascular health. Incorporating both aerobic and resistance training into one's routine can lead to significant health improvements, and personalised exercise plans can be developed to cater to individual preferences and abilities.

Moreover, stress management techniques play a crucial role in maintaining metabolic health. Practices such as mindfulness meditation, yoga, and deep-breathing exercises can help reduce stress levels, which in turn can diminish cortisol production and lower the risk of weight gain. Addressing mental health is an essential part of a holistic approach to tackling metabolic syndrome.

In conclusion, integrative approaches offer a comprehensive framework for managing metabolic syndrome effectively. By merging medical treatments with lifestyle changes, individuals can tackle the root causes of their condition. This multifaceted strategy not only improves physical health but also enhances overall well-being, demonstrating the power of synergy between medicine and lifestyle.

9

Chapter 9: Weight Management Strategies That Actually Work

Why Diets Fail: Psychology of Weight Loss

Many diets fail not only due to the physical challenges associated with weight loss but also because of the psychological barriers that individuals face. Understanding these psychological aspects is crucial, as it can illuminate why many people struggle to maintain their weight loss efforts. Emotional eating, stress, and the pressure to conform to societal standards often lead individuals to abandon their diet plans, regardless of their initial motivations.

One significant factor is the relationship between emotions and eating habits. People often turn to food for comfort during times of stress or sadness, leading to a cycle of emotional eating that can undermine diet efforts. This behaviour is not merely a lack of willpower but is rooted in deeper psychological needs for coping and self-soothing. Recognising this can help individuals develop healthier coping mechanisms that do not involve food.

Furthermore, the concept of self-efficacy plays a vital role in the psychology of weight loss. Individuals with a strong belief in their ability to succeed are more likely to stick to their diets and achieve their weight loss goals. Conversely, those who doubt their abilities may feel disheartened after setbacks, leading to a sense of failure that prompts them to give up entirely. Building confidence through small, achievable goals can help bolster self-efficacy and strengthen commitment to weight loss.

Social influences also cannot be overlooked when discussing diet failures. Peer pressure, family expectations, and cultural norms can create an environment where individuals feel they must conform to certain eating habits. When these external pressures conflict with their personal goals, it can create a sense of frustration and defeat. Understanding these influences allows individuals to navigate their social environments more effectively and advocate for their health choices.

In conclusion, the psychology of weight loss is complex and multifaceted, encompassing emotional, cognitive, and social dimensions. Acknowledging these factors can empower individuals to approach their weight loss journeys with a more informed mindset. By addressing the psychological barriers that contribute to diet failure, individuals can develop strategies that not only aid in weight loss but also promote long-term lifestyle changes.

Setting Realistic and Sustainable Goals

Setting realistic and sustainable goals is crucial for anyone looking to manage or prevent metabolic syndrome. These goals serve as a roadmap, guiding individuals toward healthier lifestyles while allowing for gradual changes that can lead to lasting results. Rather than aiming for drastic transformations, it is more effective to focus on small, achievable milestones that can be celebrated along the way. This approach not only fosters a sense of accomplishment but also encourages continued commitment to health improvement.

When setting goals, it is essential to ensure they are specific, measurable, attainable, relevant, and time-bound (SMART). For instance, instead of simply stating the desire to lose weight, an individual might set a goal to lose five kilograms within three months by incorporating regular exercise and healthier eating habits. This specificity allows for better tracking of progress and can motivate individuals to stay on course as they witness their achievements.

Moreover, sustainability is a key factor in goal-setting. Goals should align with one's lifestyle, making it easier to integrate new habits into daily routines. For example, if someone enjoys cooking, they might set a goal to try one new healthy recipe each week. By incorporating enjoyable activities, the likelihood of maintaining these healthier behaviours increases, ultimately leading to better long-term health outcomes.

It is also important to recognise the potential for setbacks. Life can be unpredictable, and some challenges may disrupt progress. Setting realistic goals should involve planning for these obstacles by identifying strategies to overcome them when they arise. This proactive approach helps individuals remain resilient and adaptable, rather than discouraged by temporary setbacks.

Finally, seeking support from friends, family, or health professionals can enhance the goal-setting process. Sharing goals with others can foster accountability and provide encouragement, which is vital for maintaining motivation. By working together, individuals can create a supportive environment that promotes the successful achievement of realistic and sustainable health goals, ultimately leading to a better understanding and management of metabolic syndrome.

Tracking Tools: Apps, Journals, and Devices

In the journey to understand and manage metabolic syndrome, tracking tools play a vital role. These tools, which include apps, journals, and devices, help individuals monitor their health metrics, diet, physical activity, and overall progress. The integration of technology in health management can empower individuals to take control of their well-being, making informed decisions based on real-time data.

The Importance of Habit Stacking and Behavior Change

Habit stacking is an effective strategy that can significantly influence behaviour change, particularly in the context of managing metabolic syndrome. By linking new habits to existing ones, individuals can create a seamless transition that makes it easier to adopt healthier behaviours. For instance, if someone already has a morning routine of brushing their teeth, they might stack a new habit, such as drinking a glass of water, immediately after. This method not only reinforces the new behaviour but also reduces the mental load associated with making changes to one's lifestyle.

Understanding the importance of habit stacking lies in its ability to create a structured approach to behaviour change. It is not merely about adding tasks but about integrating them into a daily rhythm that feels natural. This structured approach is crucial for individuals facing the challenges of metabolic syndrome, as it encourages consistent practice and reduces the likelihood of relapse into old habits. By making small, manageable changes, individuals can experience gradual improvements in their health without feeling overwhelmed.

Moreover, habit stacking promotes accountability and self-efficacy. When individuals successfully incorporate new habits into their existing routines, they build confidence in their ability to make further changes. This positive reinforcement is vital for long-term behaviour change, particularly in a health context. The journey towards managing metabolic syndrome can often feel daunting; however, small victories through habit stacking can motivate individuals to continue on their path to better health.

Incorporating habit stacking into daily life also allows for flexibility and adaptability, which are essential for sustainable behaviour change. Life is unpredictable, and individuals may face various barriers that could derail their efforts. By stacking habits, individuals can adjust their routines without completely abandoning their health goals. For example, if someone cannot exercise in the morning due to time constraints, they might stack a short workout with another established habit, such as watching television in the evening.

Ultimately, the significance of habit stacking in behaviour change extends beyond mere health management; it fosters a mindset of continuous improvement and resilience. As individuals learn to navigate the complexities of metabolic syndrome, the ability to stack habits can empower them to take control of their health. This proactive approach not only benefits physical health but also enhances overall well-being, making habit stacking a fundamental component of a healthier lifestyle.

Plateaus and How to Break Through

Plateaus in health and fitness often occur when individuals experience a period of stagnation, despite their efforts to improve their well-being. These plateaus can be particularly frustrating for those managing metabolic syndrome, as they may feel that their hard work is yielding no results. Understanding the reasons behind these plateaus is essential to breaking through them and continuing on the path to improved health.

One common reason for reaching a plateau is the body's natural adaptation to changes. When a person begins a new exercise routine or diet, their body initially responds positively by losing weight or improving metabolic markers. However, over time, the body becomes accustomed to the new regimen, leading to diminished returns. This is particularly relevant for individuals with metabolic syndrome, as their bodies may react differently due to underlying metabolic issues.

To break through these plateaus, it is vital to introduce variety into one's routine. This can mean changing the type of exercise performed, adjusting the intensity, or altering dietary habits. For example, incorporating high-intensity interval training (HIIT) can stimulate metabolic responses that may be dormant in a steady-state routine. Additionally, small modifications in diet, such as increasing protein intake or reducing carbohydrates, can also help re-ignite progress.

Another effective strategy is to reassess goals and expectations. Sometimes, unrealistic expectations can contribute to feelings of frustration when results do not align with efforts. By setting achievable short-term goals, individuals can create a sense of accomplishment and motivation that can help propel them through plateaus. It is important to celebrate small victories, as they can provide the encouragement needed to continue pursuing long-term health improvements.

Lastly, seeking support from healthcare professionals or joining support groups can play a significant role in overcoming plateaus. Engaging with others who share similar challenges can provide new insights and motivation. Healthcare providers can offer tailored advice and adjustments to management plans that can help individuals move past these stagnant periods, ensuring a continued focus on overall health and well-being.

10

Chapter 10: Women, Menopause, and Metabolic Syndrome

How Hormonal Changes Affect Weight and Metabolism

Hormonal changes play a significant role in influencing weight and metabolism, affecting individuals in various stages of life. During puberty, for example, both males and females experience surges in hormones like testosterone and oestrogen, which can lead to increased muscle mass and changes in body fat distribution. Similarly, hormonal fluctuations during the menstrual cycle can also impact appetite and energy levels, which in turn can influence weight gain or loss.

As individuals age, hormonal shifts become more pronounced, particularly during menopause for women and andropause for men. These changes can lead to a decline in metabolic rate, making it easier to gain weight and harder to lose it. The decrease in oestrogen during menopause is often associated with an increase in visceral fat, which is linked to a higher risk of metabolic syndrome.

Stress is another factor that can trigger hormonal changes, particularly the release of cortisol, which is known as the stress hormone. Elevated cortisol levels can lead to increased appetite and cravings for high-calorie foods, often resulting in weight gain. Chronic stress can also disrupt other hormones involved in metabolism, further complicating weight management efforts.

Thyroid hormones are crucial in regulating metabolism, and any imbalance can significantly affect body weight. Hypothyroidism, for instance, can slow down metabolism, leading to weight gain, fatigue, and a host of other symptoms. Conversely, hyperthyroidism can accelerate metabolism, causing weight loss and increased appetite, highlighting the delicate balance that hormones maintain in metabolic processes.

Understanding the impact of hormonal changes on weight and metabolism is essential for promoting effective weight management strategies. By recognising how different life stages and stressors influence hormonal balance, individuals can make informed decisions regarding diet and exercise. This understanding can empower individuals to take control of their weight and overall health, particularly in the context of metabolic syndrome.

HRT and Its Role (Risks vs Benefits)

Hormone Replacement Therapy (HRT) has garnered attention as a potential treatment for various health issues, particularly in the context of metabolic syndrome. This therapy aims to balance hormone levels in individuals, often focusing on those experiencing symptoms related to hormonal imbalances. While HRT may offer several benefits, it is essential to understand the associated risks to make informed decisions about its use.

The benefits of HRT can be significant, particularly for those suffering from menopausal symptoms or hormonal deficiencies. By restoring hormone levels, individuals may experience relief from symptoms such as hot flashes, night sweats, and mood swings. Additionally, HRT has been linked to improved bone density and a reduced risk of osteoporosis, which can be particularly beneficial for postmenopausal women at risk of fractures.

However, the use of HRT is not without its concerns. Research has indicated that HRT may increase the risk of certain health issues, including cardiovascular problems and certain types of cancer. It is crucial for individuals considering HRT to discuss their personal health history and risk factors with a qualified healthcare provider to assess whether the potential benefits outweigh the risks.

The decision to commence HRT should be personalised, taking into account an individual's unique health profile and lifestyle. Regular monitoring and open communication with healthcare professionals can help manage any adverse effects and ensure that the therapy remains beneficial over time. This personalised approach is vital, as it acknowledges that each person's experience with metabolic syndrome and hormonal health is different.

In conclusion, HRT can play a significant role in managing symptoms associated with hormonal imbalances and metabolic syndrome. However, it is imperative to weigh the potential benefits against the risks involved. Through informed decision-making and personalised care, individuals can navigate the complexities of HRT and make choices that promote their overall health and well-being.

Strategies Tailored to Perimenopause and Postmenopause

Perimenopause and postmenopause are significant life stages for many women, often accompanied by various physical and emotional changes. Understanding these transitions is essential for developing effective strategies to manage health, particularly regarding metabolic syndrome. The hormonal fluctuations during perimenopause can lead to weight gain, insulin resistance, and increased cardiovascular risk, making it crucial to adopt a proactive approach to health during this period.

One of the primary strategies for women in these stages is to focus on nutrition. A balanced diet rich in whole foods, including fruits, vegetables, lean proteins, and healthy fats, can help mitigate some of the symptoms associated with hormonal changes. Additionally, incorporating foods high in fibre can aid in digestion and support weight management, which is particularly important as metabolism slows down during this time.

Physical activity is another vital component of managing health during perimenopause and postmenopause. Regular exercise not only helps in maintaining a healthy weight but also improves mood and energy levels.

Women should aim for a combination of aerobic exercises, strength training, and flexibility workouts to enhance overall well-being and combat the risk factors associated with metabolic syndrome.

Stress management techniques are also essential during these life transitions. Practices such as mindfulness, yoga, and meditation can help alleviate anxiety and promote emotional balance. By incorporating these techniques into daily routines, women can better navigate the psychological challenges that may arise in conjunction with physical changes, improving their overall quality of life.

Finally, regular health screenings and consultations with healthcare professionals are crucial. Monitoring blood pressure, cholesterol levels, and glucose can help identify potential issues early on. Women should advocate for their health by discussing any symptoms or concerns with their doctors, ensuring that they receive personalised care tailored to their needs during perimenopause and postmenopause.

11

Chapter 11: Teens and Young Adults at Risk

Rising Incidence in Youth

The rising incidence of metabolic syndrome among youth is becoming an alarming trend that warrants urgent attention. Factors contributing to this increase include sedentary lifestyles, poor dietary choices, and heightened stress levels. The consequences of these lifestyle changes can lead to serious health complications, including obesity, diabetes, and cardiovascular diseases, which were once predominantly seen in adults. As young people adopt behaviours that compromise their health, the implications for public health are significant and far-reaching.

One of the primary drivers of this epidemic is the increasing prevalence of obesity in children and adolescents. The availability and marketing of high-calorie, low-nutrient foods have made unhealthy eating habits more common. Coupled with a decline in physical activity due to the rise of digital entertainment, young individuals are facing a perfect storm that fosters weight gain. This shift not only impacts their immediate health but also sets the stage for long-term metabolic issues.

Furthermore, psychological factors play a crucial role in the rising incidence of metabolic syndrome in youth. Stress, anxiety, and depression can lead to emotional eating and a lack of motivation to engage in physical activity. The pressures of modern life, compounded by social media influences, can create a cycle where unhealthy coping mechanisms become the norm. It is essential to address these mental health challenges to combat the physical health crisis effectively.

Education and awareness are key components in reversing this trend. Schools and communities must work together to promote healthier lifestyle choices among the younger population. Initiatives that encourage physical activity, provide nutritional education, and support mental well-being can make a significant difference. By fostering an environment that prioritises health, we can empower youth to make informed decisions about their lifestyle.

In conclusion, the rising incidence of metabolic syndrome in youth is a multifaceted issue that requires comprehensive strategies for prevention and intervention. A collaborative effort involving families, schools, and healthcare providers is essential to address the root causes of this epidemic. By understanding and tackling the factors contributing to metabolic syndrome, we can help ensure a healthier future for the next generation.

Screen Time, Processed Foods, and Sedentary Habits

In today's world, screen time has become an integral part of daily life, with many individuals spending hours each day in front of various screens. This includes not only television but also smartphones, tablets, and computers. Such excessive screen exposure is often linked to a range of health issues, including obesity and metabolic syndrome, as it encourages a sedentary lifestyle that reduces physical activity levels significantly.

Processed foods are another significant factor contributing to the rise of metabolic syndrome. These products are typically high in sugar, unhealthy fats, and preservatives, which can lead to weight gain and insulin resistance. The convenience of processed foods is appealing, but their long-term consumption can have detrimental effects on metabolic health, making it crucial to understand their impact and seek healthier alternatives.

Sedentary habits, often exacerbated by increased screen time and reliance on processed foods, are prevalent in modern society. Many people find themselves leading a lifestyle that involves prolonged sitting, whether at work or during leisure activities. This lack of movement not only contributes to weight gain but also increases the risk of developing chronic conditions associated with metabolic syndrome, such as type 2 diabetes and cardiovascular disease.

To combat the adverse effects of screen time, processed foods, and sedentary habits, individuals can adopt simple yet effective strategies. Incorporating regular physical activity into daily routines, such as walking or cycling, can significantly improve metabolic health. Additionally, making conscious dietary choices by prioritising whole, unprocessed foods can help to mitigate the risks associated with metabolic syndrome and promote overall well-being.

Raising awareness about the dangers of excessive screen time, the consumption of processed foods, and the importance of staying active is essential for public health. By fostering a culture of healthy living, individuals can be empowered to make informed choices that positively impact their metabolic health. Ultimately, understanding the interplay between lifestyle choices and metabolic syndrome is vital for achieving long-term health goals and enhancing quality of life.

Family-Based Interventions

Family-based interventions represent a crucial strategy in addressing metabolic syndrome, as they leverage the power of collective support and shared lifestyle changes. When families engage in healthier habits together, they create an environment that promotes better nutrition and increased physical activity. This collaborative approach not only enhances individual motivation but also strengthens family bonds, making the journey towards better health a shared experience.

One effective model for family-based interventions is the incorporation of family meals. Research shows that families who eat together are more likely to consume nutritious foods and establish positive eating patterns. Regular family meals can serve as a platform for discussing health, encouraging children and adolescents to make better food choices and reducing the likelihood of developing obesity and related metabolic conditions.

Moreover, physical activity is another area where family-based interventions can have a significant impact. Families that engage in physical activities together, such as walking, cycling, or playing sports, not only improve their fitness levels but also nurture a sense of teamwork and enjoyment. This shared commitment to an active lifestyle helps to instil lifelong habits in younger family members, reducing their risk of metabolic syndrome later in life.

Education and awareness also play a pivotal role in family-based interventions. By providing families with information on the risk factors and consequences of metabolic syndrome, they can make informed decisions about their lifestyle choices. Workshops and group sessions can empower families with practical skills, such as meal planning and cooking healthy recipes, thereby equipping them with the tools necessary for lasting change.

In conclusion, family-based interventions offer a holistic approach to combating metabolic syndrome by fostering a supportive environment for healthy lifestyle changes. When families work together to improve their habits, they not only enhance their individual health outcomes but also strengthen their relationships. This collective effort is vital in addressing the growing prevalence of metabolic syndrome in society today.

Preventing Long-Term Health Complications

Preventing long-term health complications associated with metabolic syndrome requires a multifaceted approach that encompasses lifestyle modifications, regular health screenings, and education. Individuals must prioritise maintaining a healthy weight through balanced nutrition and consistent physical activity. These changes not only aid in managing existing conditions but also serve as a proactive measure against the onset of more serious health issues, such as diabetes and cardiovascular disease.

Incorporating a diet rich in fruits, vegetables, whole grains, and lean proteins is essential. Reducing the intake of processed foods and sugars can significantly lower the risk factors linked to metabolic syndrome. Additionally, regular physical activity—ideally, at least 150 minutes of moderate aerobic exercise weekly—can enhance insulin sensitivity and contribute to weight management, further mitigating risks.

Regular health screenings play a crucial role in early detection and management of metabolic syndrome. Blood pressure, cholesterol levels, and blood glucose should be monitored consistently. These screenings allow for timely interventions, which can prevent complications such as heart disease and stroke. Individuals should work closely with healthcare professionals to tailor their health plans based on personal risk factors and family history.

Education about metabolic syndrome is vital for both patients and healthcare providers. By understanding the condition and its implications, individuals are more likely to engage in preventative behaviours. Community programmes and workshops can foster a supportive environment where one learns about healthy lifestyle choices and the importance of regular check-ups, ultimately leading to better health outcomes.

Lastly, managing stress is often an overlooked yet critical aspect of preventing long-term health complications. Chronic stress can exacerbate the effects of metabolic syndrome, making it essential to incorporate stress-reducing practices such as mindfulness, yoga, or regular social interactions. By addressing both physical and mental health, individuals can significantly improve their overall well-being and reduce the risk of serious health complications associated with metabolic syndrome.

12

Chapter 12: Reclaiming Health – Case Studies and Real-World Stories

Success Stories with Lifestyle Change

Success stories of individuals who have embraced lifestyle changes provide powerful motivation for others facing metabolic syndrome. These narratives highlight the transformative power of small, consistent adjustments to daily routines. By sharing their journeys, these individuals not only inspire hope but also demonstrate that achieving better health is possible with dedication and perseverance.

One compelling example is that of Sarah, a 45-year-old woman who struggled with obesity and related health issues. After being diagnosed with metabolic syndrome, she decided to make significant changes to her diet and exercise routine. By incorporating whole foods and regular physical activity, Sarah lost over 30 kilograms and improved her blood sugar levels. Her story exemplifies how determination can lead to substantial health improvements.

Similarly, John, a 50-year-old man with a family history of diabetes, realised the importance of taking control of his health. After attending a wellness seminar, he adopted a Mediterranean diet and began walking daily. Within months, John noticed a remarkable decrease in his cholesterol levels and increased energy. His success highlights not only the impact of dietary choices but also the role of community support in fostering lasting change.

Moreover, the journey of Lisa, a 38-year-old mother, illustrates the significance of mental well-being alongside physical health. Faced with stress and weight gain, Lisa sought mindfulness practices such as yoga and meditation, which complemented her nutritional changes. As a result, she experienced improved mental clarity and emotional resilience, reinforcing the idea that lifestyle changes can be holistic in nature.

These success stories collectively emphasise that lifestyle modifications are not just about weight loss but encompass a broader spectrum of health benefits. They inspire others to consider their own health journeys, proving that with the right mindset and support, overcoming the challenges of metabolic syndrome is achievable for everyone.

Overcoming Setbacks and Relapses

Overcoming setbacks and relapses is a crucial aspect of managing metabolic syndrome. Individuals often face challenges that can impede their progress, such as dietary lapses or periods of inactivity. Understanding that these setbacks are a natural part of any health journey is vital. Instead of viewing them as failures, individuals should recognise them as opportunities to learn and adapt their strategies for better outcomes in the future.

One effective approach to overcoming setbacks is to establish a supportive network. Engaging with friends, family, or support groups can provide the encouragement needed to stay motivated. Sharing experiences and challenges with others can foster a sense of community and accountability. This support can be instrumental in helping individuals navigate through tough times and maintain focus on their health goals.

Additionally, setting realistic and achievable goals can mitigate feelings of discouragement when setbacks occur. It is important for individuals to break down their larger objectives into smaller, manageable steps. Celebrating these small victories can build confidence and reinforce positive behaviours. This incremental approach allows for flexibility, enabling individuals to adjust their plans without losing sight of their overall health aspirations.

Practising self-compassion is another vital element in overcoming setbacks. Individuals must learn to forgive themselves for any missteps and avoid harsh self-criticism. Acknowledging that everyone experiences setbacks can alleviate feelings of isolation and despair. By treating themselves with kindness, individuals can cultivate a more positive mindset, which is essential for long-term success in managing metabolic syndrome.

Finally, it is crucial to remain adaptable in the face of challenges. Life can be unpredictable, and circumstances may change, requiring individuals to reassess and modify their health strategies. Embracing flexibility and being open to trying new approaches can lead to discovering effective methods for managing metabolic syndrome. Ultimately, resilience and determination in overcoming setbacks will significantly contribute to an individual's journey towards better health and well-being.

Role of Support Networks, Coaching, and Accountability

Support networks play a crucial role in managing metabolic syndrome, as they provide the necessary emotional and practical assistance individuals often need. Friends, family, and peer groups can create an encouraging environment where individuals feel motivated to adopt healthier lifestyles. This support can lead to better adherence to dietary changes and exercise routines, significantly impacting overall health outcomes.

Coaching is another vital element in the journey towards better health. A qualified coach can offer personalised advice and strategies tailored to an individual's specific needs and circumstances. This guidance not only helps in setting realistic goals but also in developing actionable plans to achieve them. Coaches often serve as a source of accountability, ensuring that individuals stay committed to their health objectives.

Accountability is paramount when it comes to sustaining lifestyle changes. Having someone to report progress to can foster a sense of responsibility, pushing individuals to remain consistent with their efforts. Whether it's a coach, a support group, or even an app that tracks progress, accountability mechanisms help reinforce positive behaviours and discourage relapse into unhealthy habits.

Incorporating these elements into a lifestyle change programme can create a comprehensive approach to tackling metabolic syndrome. It is not merely about individual effort; rather, it is about building a community where support and encouragement are at the forefront. This collective effort can lead to more sustainable results and improved overall well-being.

Ultimately, understanding the role of support networks, coaching, and accountability is essential for anyone looking to manage or prevent metabolic syndrome. By recognising the importance of these components, individuals can harness their potential to create lasting changes in their health and lifestyle, leading to a better quality of life.

13

Chapter 13: Designing Your Personal Metabolic Reset Plan

Checklist: Where Do You Stand?

Understanding where you stand in relation to metabolic syndrome is crucial for taking proactive steps towards better health. This checklist serves as a self-assessment tool, allowing you to identify any potential risk factors associated with this condition. By evaluating your lifestyle, family history, and personal health metrics, you can gain valuable insights into your current state of well-being.

Firstly, consider your body measurements. Pay attention to your waist circumference, as excess abdominal fat is a significant indicator of metabolic syndrome. Additionally, assess your body mass index (BMI) to determine if you fall within a healthy range. These measurements can provide a clear picture of your risk level and guide your next steps.

Next, evaluate your diet and physical activity levels. A diet high in processed foods, sugars, and unhealthy fats can contribute to metabolic syndrome. Conversely, regular physical activity can help mitigate these risks. Reflect on your eating habits and exercise routine, noting any areas where improvements can be made to promote a healthier lifestyle.

Another important factor to consider is your blood pressure and cholesterol levels. High blood pressure and elevated cholesterol are key components of metabolic syndrome. Check your recent health records or consult with a healthcare provider to understand where you stand regarding these metrics. Keeping track of these numbers can empower you to make informed decisions about your health.

Finally, remember that family history plays a significant role in your risk for developing metabolic syndrome. If you have relatives with conditions such as diabetes or heart disease, it's essential to take these factors into account. By acknowledging your genetic predisposition, you can take proactive measures to monitor and improve your health, ensuring you stay on the right path toward well-being.

4-Week Reset Program Template

The 4-Week Reset Program is designed as a structured approach to address metabolic syndrome by encouraging participants to adopt healthier lifestyles. Throughout these four weeks, individuals will focus on improving their diet, increasing physical activity, and managing stress levels. Each week builds upon the last, providing a gradual ramp-up to more significant changes that can lead to lasting habits and an overall healthier lifestyle.

In the first week, participants will begin by eliminating processed foods, sugars, and unhealthy fats. This foundational step is crucial as it helps to clear the body of harmful substances and sets the stage for healthier eating. Instead, individuals will be encouraged to consume whole foods, such as fruits, vegetables, lean proteins, and whole grains, which provide essential nutrients and support metabolic health.

The second week introduces the concept of portion control and mindful eating. Participants will learn to listen to their bodies and recognise hunger and fullness cues. This week also focuses on meal prepping, which can help individuals stay on track with their dietary goals. By planning meals in advance, it becomes easier to avoid unhealthy temptations and make better food choices.

As the program progresses into the third week, physical activity becomes the central theme. Individuals will be encouraged to incorporate at least 150 minutes of moderate exercise into their weekly routine. This can include activities such as brisk walking, swimming, or cycling. Regular exercise not only aids in weight management but also improves cardiovascular health and insulin sensitivity, both of which are critical factors in managing metabolic syndrome.

Finally, the fourth week emphasises stress management and the importance of mental well-being. Participants will be introduced to various techniques such as mindfulness, meditation, and deep breathing exercises. Managing stress is vital as it can negatively impact eating habits and physical health. By the end of the program, individuals will have developed a comprehensive toolkit to help them maintain a healthier lifestyle and reduce their risk of metabolic syndrome.

Monitoring Progress with SMART Goals

Monitoring progress is a crucial aspect of managing metabolic syndrome, and using SMART goals can significantly enhance this process. SMART stands for Specific, Measurable, Achievable, Relevant, and Time-bound. By setting SMART goals, individuals can create a clear framework that helps them stay focused and motivated in their journey towards better health. This structured approach allows for the identification of specific targets, such as reducing waist circumference or lowering blood pressure, which are essential in combating metabolic syndrome.

The first step in establishing SMART goals is to make them specific. Instead of vague aims like 'I want to lose weight,' a specific goal would be 'I want to lose 5 kilograms in three months.' This clarity helps individuals understand exactly what they need to achieve. Furthermore, being specific allows for better planning and the formulation of strategies to reach these targets effectively.

Next, goals must be measurable to track progress accurately. This could involve using tools like a scale, measuring tape, or health apps that record daily activity levels. Having measurable goals enables individuals to see their advancements and adjust their strategies as needed. For example, if the goal is to exercise for 30 minutes five times a week, logging workouts can provide tangible evidence of commitment and improvement.

Achievable goals are vital to maintain motivation. It is essential that the targets set are realistic and attainable within a given timeframe. Overly ambitious goals can lead to frustration and a sense of failure, which may ultimately discourage individuals from continuing their efforts. Setting smaller, incremental goals can lead to sustained success and a greater sense of accomplishment, reinforcing positive behaviours.

Finally, ensuring that goals are relevant and time-bound helps align the individual's health objectives with their lifestyle and commitments. A relevant goal could be to improve overall cardiovascular health through specific dietary changes. By establishing a deadline, such as completing a health assessment in six months, individuals can create a sense of urgency that encourages them to stay on track. Monitoring progress with SMART goals not only promotes accountability but also fosters a proactive approach to managing metabolic syndrome effectively.

Staying Consistent for Life

Consistency is the cornerstone of any successful lifestyle change, particularly when addressing metabolic syndrome. Establishing a routine that incorporates healthy eating, regular physical activity, and stress management can significantly improve one's overall health. It is essential to understand that making these changes is not merely a temporary fix but a lifelong commitment. Only by embracing consistency can individuals hope to see lasting results and effectively manage their metabolic health.

Building habits takes time, and it is crucial to approach this journey with patience. Incremental changes are often more sustainable than drastic overhauls. For instance, starting with small, manageable dietary adjustments, such as incorporating more fruits and vegetables into meals, can pave the way for more significant improvements. Regular check-ins with oneself can also help maintain focus and motivation, ensuring that one remains on track with their health goals.

Support from family and friends plays a vital role in maintaining consistency. Sharing goals with loved ones can create a sense of accountability and encouragement. Joining support groups or community initiatives can also provide additional motivation and resources. Engaging with others who share similar health objectives can foster a supportive environment that nurtures perseverance and commitment to healthy living.

Moreover, it is important to celebrate small victories along the way. Acknowledging progress, no matter how minor, can boost morale and reinforce the desire to continue. This positive reinforcement can be pivotal in overcoming obstacles and setbacks that may arise. Remembering why one embarked on this journey in the first place can also serve as a powerful motivator during challenging times.

In conclusion, staying consistent for life requires dedication, patience, and support. By adopting a proactive mindset and embracing gradual changes, individuals can significantly impact their metabolic health. The journey may be challenging, but the rewards of consistent effort will lead to a healthier, more fulfilling life. Ultimately, the goal is not just to manage metabolic syndrome but to thrive in all aspects of life, making health a priority for years to come.

14

Briefing Document: Metabolic Syndrome: Reclaiming Health

Purpose: This briefing document summarizes the key themes, ideas, and facts presented in "Metabolic Syndrome: Reclaiming Health," offering a comprehensive overview of the condition, its causes, risks, and strategies for management and reversal.

I. Understanding Metabolic Syndrome: Definition, Prevalence, and Diagnostic Criteria

Metabolic Syndrome is presented as "a cluster of conditions that increase the risk of heart disease, stroke, and diabetes." Its prevalence is "rising in recent years, largely due to lifestyle changes such as poor diet and physical inactivity." Many individuals are unaware they have it due to "subtle or non-existent" symptoms. Early identification through "regular health screenings and awareness of the risk factors" is crucial.

Key Diagnostic Criteria (requiring a combination of these factors):

- **Waist Circumference:** Reflects central obesity. "For men, a waist measurement of more than 102 cm (40 inches) and for women, more than 88 cm (35 inches) indicates a higher risk."

- **Blood Pressure:** "Elevated blood pressure, defined as a reading of 130/85 mmHg or higher."
- **Lipid Levels:Triglycerides:** "150 mg/dL or higher."
- **HDL Cholesterol:** "Less than 40 mg/dL for men and less than 50 mg/dL for women."
- **Glucose Levels:** "A fasting glucose level of 100 mg/dL or higher."

II. Long-Term Health Risks and Development Over Time

Metabolic syndrome "significantly increase[s] the risk of developing serious health issues over time," including "cardiovascular diseases, type 2 diabetes, and other chronic health problems." These can "ultimately diminish their quality of life."

How it Develops:

- It "develops gradually over time, influenced by a multitude of factors including genetics, lifestyle, and environmental elements."
- Initially, "subtle changes in body composition and metabolic processes are already underway," often involving "accumulation of visceral fat and insulin resistance."
- "As time progresses, the effects... become more pronounced," with "insidious" changes in blood pressure, cholesterol, and glucose.
- **Key Drivers:** "Lifestyle choices such as diet and physical activity. Poor dietary habits, characterised by high sugar and fat intake, coupled with a sedentary lifestyle, can exacerbate the condition."
- "Psychological factors such as stress and lack of sleep can also play a significant role."

III. The Underlying Causes of Metabolic Syndrome

The source identifies several core causes contributing to metabolic syndrome:

- **Insulin Resistance:** "The core problem... occurs when the body's cells become less responsive to insulin." This leads to "higher blood sugar levels and an increased risk of type 2 diabetes," and forces the body to "store excess fat, particularly in the abdominal region."

- **Visceral Fat and Inflammation:** Visceral fat (abdominal fat around organs) is "an active endocrine organ that can release various inflammatory markers into the bloodstream." This presence is "closely linked to chronic inflammation in the body" and "can disrupt the normal functioning of insulin, leading to insulin resistance."
- **Genetics and Family History:** "Genetics play a significant role... Individuals with a family history of metabolic disorders are often more susceptible." "Epigenetics" (environmental influence on gene expression) also plays a role, meaning "lifestyle choices... can either exacerbate or alleviate genetic predispositions."
- **Hormonal Imbalance:Leptin:** "Satiety hormone." Leptin resistance can occur in obesity, leading to "increased appetite and weight gain."
- **Cortisol:** "Stress hormone." "Chronic elevation due to prolonged stress can lead to increased fat accumulation, particularly in the abdominal area."
- **Ghrelin:** "Hunger hormone." "Elevated levels... can contribute to overeating and obesity."
- **Sedentary Lifestyle and Poor Diet Patterns:** These are deeply intertwined. "Lack of activity can lead to a variety of health issues, including obesity, cardiovascular diseases, and ultimately, metabolic syndrome." Poor diets are "high in processed foods, sugars, and unhealthy fats." This creates a "vicious cycle that is difficult to break."

IV. Risk Factors and Early Warning Signs

Specific populations and conditions are highlighted as being "most at risk":

- **Family History:** Of diabetes or cardiovascular disease.
- **Age:** "As people get older, the likelihood of developing conditions such as obesity, hypertension, and insulin resistance rises."

- **Lifestyle Choices:** "Sedentary behaviour, poor diet, and excessive alcohol consumption."
- **Gender:** "Men are generally at a higher risk compared to women, particularly in terms of abdominal obesity. However, post-menopausal women may experience an increased risk due to hormonal changes."
- **Ethnicity:** "Hispanic, African American, and Native American populations."
- **Associated Conditions:Pre-diabetes:** "Often a precursor to type 2 diabetes, characterised by elevated blood glucose levels." It is "a warning sign that should not be ignored."
- **Polycystic Ovary Syndrome (PCOS):** "Closely linked to insulin resistance," leading to "irregular menstrual cycles, weight gain, and fertility issues."
- **Fatty Liver Disease (NAFLD):** "Characterised by the accumulation of fat in liver cells." It "often coexists with pre-diabetes and PCOS" and "can signal underlying insulin resistance." It acts as a "crucial red flag."

Monitoring Tools:

- **Waist-to-Hip Ratio (WHR):** "A crucial measurement that helps assess body fat distribution." A higher WHR is linked to increased risk. "A WHR of 0.85 or less is typically considered healthy for women, while a ratio of 0.90 or less is deemed acceptable for men."
- **Blood Tests:Fasting Glucose:** "Measures the sugar level in the blood after an overnight fast." Elevated levels may indicate insulin resistance.
- **HbA1c:** "Reflects average blood glucose levels over the past two to three months." Useful for diagnosing prediabetes (5.7% to 6.4%) and diabetes (6.5% or higher).
- **Triglycerides (TG):** "High levels... can contribute to the hardening of arteries." "Above 150 mg/dL is considered high."
- **High-density lipoprotein (HDL) cholesterol:** "Good' cholesterol." "Less than 40 mg/dL in men and less than 50 mg/dL in women is considered low."

V. Nutrition for Reversing Metabolic Syndrome

Nutrition is a cornerstone of management:

- **Carbohydrate Quality over Quantity:** "High-quality carbohydrates, such as whole grains, fruits, and vegetables, provide... vital nutrients and fibre." "Low-quality carbohydrates, often found in processed foods, can lead to spikes in blood sugar and ultimately contribute to metabolic syndrome." Emphasize "complex carbohydrates" and low-glycemic index (GI) foods.
- **Low-Glycemic and Anti-Inflammatory Eating:** Focus on foods with "minimal impact on blood sugar levels," and those "rich in antioxidants, such as berries, leafy greens, and nuts," and "Omega-3 fatty acids." "Hydration is another key aspect."
- **Protein and Healthy Fats for Satiety and Insulin Balance:Protein:** Promotes "greater feeling of fullness" by influencing appetite hormones, curbing hunger and reducing overeating.
- **Healthy Fats:** "Provide a more stable source of energy" and "contribute to the absorption of fat-soluble vitamins." They lead to "a more balanced blood sugar response."
- This emphasis naturally reduces "processed foods high in sugars and unhealthy fats."
- **Sample Meal Plans & Grocery List:** Practical tools for incorporating whole foods, lean proteins, healthy fats, and avoiding processed items.
- **Addressing Sugar Addiction and Emotional Eating:** "Significant factors contributing to metabolic syndrome." Requires "recognising triggers for sugar cravings," "educating oneself on nutrition," utilizing "support systems," and "seeking professional help" when needed.

VI. Intermittent Fasting and Time-Restricted Eating

These dietary patterns are presented as effective strategies:

- **How it Works:** By creating periods of fasting, these methods can lead to "weight loss and improved metabolic health," particularly by helping to "reduce insulin resistance."

- **Different Methods:16:8:** "Fasting for 16 hours each day and eating within an 8-hour window."
- **5:2:** "Consume a normal diet for five days of the week and restrict calorie intake to about 500-600 calories on two non-consecutive days."
- **Eat-Stop-Eat:** "A 24-hour fast once or twice a week."
- **Who Should/Shouldn't Try It:** Generally beneficial for those at risk (obesity, hypertension, diabetes). Caution is advised for "individuals with pre-existing health issues, such as heart disease, kidney problems, or severe mental health conditions." Consultation with healthcare professionals is paramount.
- **Common Pitfalls:** "Misunderstanding of what constitutes a healthy lifestyle," "rely[ing] on quick fixes or fad diets," "lack of awareness about the importance of stress management," and overlooking "social support." Starting safely involves "personalised plans that focus on gradual, sustainable changes" and "realistic expectations."

VII. Exercise and Physical Activity

Exercise is a critical intervention:

- **Benefits:** "Improving insulin sensitivity and promoting fat burning." It "significantly decrease[s] the risk of type 2 diabetes" and aids in "weight management and reducing body fat percentage."
- **Aerobic vs. Resistance Training:Aerobic Training:** (walking, running, swimming) "Essential for burning calories and fat," improving cardiovascular health, enhancing insulin sensitivity, and lowering blood pressure.
- **Resistance Training:** (weights, bands, bodyweight) "Build muscle strength, endurance, and mass," increasing metabolic rate, improving body composition, and supporting better glucose metabolism.
- A combination of both is "particularly effective."
- **NEAT (Non-Exercise Activity Thermogenesis):** "Energy expenditure that

occurs during daily activities that are not classified as formal exercise." Simple actions like "taking the stairs" or "walking during phone calls" can "significantly increase daily calorie expenditure."

- **Building a Weekly Routine:** Focus on consistency, aiming for "at least 150 minutes of moderate aerobic exercise or 75 minutes of vigorous activity each week," alongside planned nutrition and stress management.
- **Managing Exercise with Obesity/Joint Pain:** Requires "a thoughtful approach that prioritises safety and effectiveness." Recommended are "low-impact activities such as swimming, cycling, and walking," along with flexibility and strength training. Encouraging individuals to "listen to their bodies" and seeking professional guidance is key.

VIII. Stress, Sleep, and Hormonal Balance

These factors are deeply intertwined with metabolic health:

- **The Cortisol Connection:** "Stress hormone." "Chronic stress can lead to prolonged elevated levels of cortisol," which "can lead to increased appetite and cravings for unhealthy foods... result in weight gain, particularly around the abdomen." It may also "promote insulin resistance."
- **How Sleep Affects Weight and Metabolism:** "Insufficient sleep can lead to hormonal imbalances, particularly in leptin and ghrelin," promoting increased ghrelin (hunger) and reduced leptin (fullness). "Poor sleep quality is linked to reduced insulin sensitivity."
- **Tools for Better Sleep Hygiene:** "Creating a consistent sleep schedule, making your sleeping environment conducive to rest, and practising relaxation techniques."
- **Stress Management:Mindfulness:** "Focus on the present moment, helping to reduce anxiety."
- **Cognitive Behavioural Therapy (CBT):** "Focuses on identifying and challenging negative thought patterns."
- **Breathing Techniques:** "Activate the body's relaxation response, reducing tension."

- Combining these offers a "comprehensive approach."

IX. The Role of Medications and Supplements

Medications and supplements can support, but not replace, lifestyle changes:

- **Metformin:** "First-line medication... improves insulin sensitivity and reducing hepatic glucose production," also contributing to weight management.
- **GLP-1 Agonists (e.g., Ozempic, Semaglutide):** "Mimic the incretin hormone," enhancing insulin secretion, promoting weight loss, and improving glycemic control. They also have "cardiovascular benefits."
- **Supplements:Omega-3:** "Anti-inflammatory properties and their ability to improve cardiovascular health," lowering triglycerides.
- **Berberine:** "Help regulate blood sugar levels," enhancing insulin sensitivity and improving lipid profiles.
- **Magnesium:** "Vital role in numerous biochemical reactions... including those involved in glucose metabolism and blood pressure regulation."
- **Vitamin D:** "Linked low levels... to increased risks of obesity, insulin resistance, and cardiovascular disorders."
- **Risks of Relying Solely on Pills:** Can lead to "neglecting essential components such as diet, exercise, and stress management." Risks include "side effects," "financial burden," and negative "psychological impact," fostering dependency.
- **Integrative Approaches:** "Focus on the synergy between traditional medicine and lifestyle changes." This "combining medical treatments with lifestyle modifications" leads to "better overall health outcomes."

X. Weight Management Strategies That Actually Work

Beyond specific interventions, successful weight management requires a holistic approach:

- **Why Diets Fail: Psychology of Weight Loss:** Failure often stems from "psychological barriers" like "emotional eating, stress, and the pressure to conform to societal standards." "Self-efficacy" and "social influences" are crucial.
- **Setting Realistic and Sustainable Goals:** Goals should be "Specific, Measurable, Attainable, Relevant, and Time-bound (SMART)." Focus on "small, achievable milestones."
- **Tracking Tools:** "Apps, journals, and devices" help monitor "health metrics, diet, physical activity, and overall progress."
- **Importance of Habit Stacking and Behavior Change:** "Linking new habits to existing ones" creates "a seamless transition." This "reduces the mental load" and promotes "accountability and self-efficacy."
- **Plateaus and How to Break Through:** Plateaus occur due to "the body's natural adaptation." Solutions include introducing "variety into one's routine" (e.g., changing exercise type/intensity, altering diet), "re-assess[ing] goals and expectations," and "seeking support from health-care professionals or joining support groups."

XI. Specific Considerations for Different Demographics

Metabolic syndrome manifests differently and requires tailored approaches for various groups:

- **Women, Menopause, and Metabolic Syndrome:Hormonal Changes:** "As individuals age, hormonal shifts become more pronounced, particularly during menopause for women." The "decrease in oestrogen during menopause is often associated with an increase in visceral fat."
- **HRT (Hormone Replacement Therapy):** Can offer "relief from symptoms" and "improved bone density." However, "may increase the risk of certain health issues, including cardiovascular problems and certain types of cancer." Decision should be "personalised."
- **Tailored Strategies:** Focus on "nutrition" (balanced diet), "physical activity" (aerobic, strength, flexibility), "stress management techniques,"

and "regular health screenings."

- **Teens and Young Adults at Risk:Rising Incidence:** "An alarming trend" due to "sedentary lifestyles, poor dietary choices, and heightened stress levels." Leads to "obesity, diabetes, and cardiovascular diseases, which were once predominantly seen in adults."
- **Contributing Factors:** "Excessive screen exposure," "processed foods," and "sedentary habits."
- **Family-Based Interventions:** "Leverage the power of collective support and shared lifestyle changes." Includes "incorporation of family meals" and "physical activity together." "Education and awareness" are pivotal.
- **Preventing Long-Term Complications:** "Multifaceted approach that encompasses lifestyle modifications, regular health screenings, and education."

XII. Reclaiming Health - Empowerment and Support

The document emphasizes the power of individuals to take control of their health:

- **Success Stories with Lifestyle Change:** "Provide powerful motivation," demonstrating that "achieving better health is possible with dedication and perseverance."
- **Overcoming Setbacks and Relapses:** Acknowledge them as "a natural part of any health journey." Strategies include "supportive network," "setting realistic and achievable goals," "practising self-compassion," and "remain[ing] adaptable."
- **Role of Support Networks, Coaching, and Accountability:** These are "crucial" elements for "personalised advice," "setting realistic goals," and ensuring "better adherence to dietary changes and exercise routines."
- **Designing Your Personal Metabolic Reset Plan:Checklist: Where Do You Stand?:** A self-assessment tool covering "body measurements (waist circumference, BMI)," "diet and physical activity levels," "blood pressure and cholesterol levels," and "family history."

- **4-Week Reset Program Template:** A structured approach starting with "eliminating processed foods," then "portion control and mindful eating," followed by "physical activity," and finally "stress management and mental well-being."
- **Monitoring Progress with SMART Goals:** (Specific, Measurable, Achievable, Relevant, Time-bound) provides a "clear framework that helps them stay focused and motivated."
- **Staying Consistent for Life:** "The cornerstone of any successful lifestyle change." Requires "patience," "incremental changes," "support from family and friends," and "celebrating small victories." The ultimate goal is "not just to manage metabolic syndrome but to thrive in all aspects of life."

15

FAQ

What is Metabolic Syndrome and why is it important to understand?

Metabolic syndrome is a collection of interconnected conditions that significantly elevate an individual's risk for serious health issues such as heart disease, stroke, and type 2 diabetes. It is characterized by a combination of high blood pressure, elevated blood sugar levels, excess body fat concentrated around the waist (visceral fat), and abnormal cholesterol levels. Understanding this syndrome is critical because its prevalence is increasing globally due to lifestyle factors like poor diet and physical inactivity. Many individuals may be unaware they have it due to subtle or absent symptoms, making regular health screenings and awareness of risk factors crucial for early identification and management. Unaddressed, metabolic syndrome can lead to severe and long-term health complications, diminishing quality of life.

What are the key diagnostic criteria for Metabolic Syndrome?

The diagnosis of metabolic syndrome relies on a combination of specific health indicators. These include:

- **Waist Circumference:** Reflecting central obesity, a measurement over 102 cm (40 inches) for men and over 88 cm (35 inches) for women indicates a higher risk.
- **Blood Pressure:** Elevated readings of 130/85 mmHg or higher are a key criterion.
- **Lipid Levels:** Abnormalities include triglyceride levels of 150 mg/dL or higher, and low HDL cholesterol (less than 40 mg/dL for men and less than 50 mg/dL for women).
- **Glucose Levels:** A fasting glucose level of 100 mg/dL or higher is indicative of impaired glucose metabolism.

Meeting a certain number of these criteria typically leads to a diagnosis of metabolic syndrome, allowing for proactive steps towards management.

What are the underlying causes of Metabolic Syndrome?

Metabolic syndrome develops over time due to a complex interplay of genetic, lifestyle, and environmental factors. Key underlying causes include:

- **Insulin Resistance:** This is considered the core problem, where the body's cells become less responsive to insulin, leading to elevated blood sugar and increased fat storage, especially visceral fat.
- **Visceral Fat and Inflammation:** Excess visceral fat (fat around internal organs) is metabolically active and releases pro-inflammatory cytokines, contributing to chronic inflammation and exacerbating insulin resistance.
- **Genetics and Family History:** Individuals with a family history of metabolic disorders are more susceptible due to inherited traits, though lifestyle choices can influence gene expression (epigenetics).
- **Hormonal Imbalance:** Dysregulation of hormones like leptin (satiety hormone), cortisol (stress hormone), and ghrelin (hunger hormone) can disrupt appetite regulation, fat accumulation, and stress response, all contributing to metabolic dysfunction.
- **Sedentary Lifestyle and Poor Diet Patterns:** A lack of physical activity

combined with diets high in processed foods, sugars, and unhealthy fats are major contributors, creating a vicious cycle of weight gain and metabolic disruption.

What lifestyle modifications are crucial for managing and potentially reversing Metabolic Syndrome?

Lifestyle modifications are paramount for managing and reversing metabolic syndrome, often proving more effective than medication alone. Key strategies include:

- **Nutrition:** Adopting a balanced diet prioritizing high-quality, complex carbohydrates (whole grains, fruits, vegetables) over refined ones, focusing on low-glycemic and anti-inflammatory foods. Emphasizing lean proteins and healthy fats helps promote satiety and insulin balance, reducing cravings and stabilizing blood sugar. Sample meal plans and grocery lists can aid in practical implementation, and addressing sugar addiction and emotional eating is crucial.
- **Physical Activity:** Regular exercise significantly improves insulin sensitivity and promotes fat burning. A combination of aerobic training (e.g., walking, swimming) for cardiovascular health and resistance training (e.g., weights, bodyweight) for muscle building and metabolic rate enhancement is recommended. Increasing Non-Exercise Activity Thermogenesis (NEAT) by integrating more movement into daily life also contributes.
- **Weight Management:** Losing excess weight, especially visceral fat, is a vital step. This is supported by dietary changes and increased physical activity.
- **Stress Management and Sleep:** Chronic stress elevates cortisol levels, negatively impacting metabolism and promoting fat storage. Techniques like mindfulness, CBT, and breathing exercises can help. Adequate and quality sleep is also crucial, as insufficient sleep disrupts hormones regulating appetite and metabolism, leading to reduced insulin sensitivity

and weight gain. Tools for better sleep hygiene are important for overall metabolic health.

How can intermittent fasting or time-restricted eating support metabolic health?

Intermittent fasting (IF) or time-restricted eating involves cycles of eating and fasting, which can significantly benefit metabolic health, particularly for managing metabolic syndrome. These methods work by allowing the body to enter a state where it burns stored fat for energy and improves insulin sensitivity. Common methods include:

- **16:8 Method:** Fasting for 16 hours and eating within an 8-hour window daily.
- **5:2 Method:** Eating normally for five days and restricting calorie intake to 500-600 calories on two non-consecutive days.
- **Eat-Stop-Eat:** A 24-hour fast once or twice a week.

These approaches can promote weight loss, reduce insulin resistance, improve blood sugar control, and lower inflammation, all of which are key factors in metabolic syndrome. However, it's crucial to consult a healthcare professional before starting IF, especially for individuals with pre-existing conditions, as certain populations (e.g., pregnant women, individuals with severe health issues) should avoid it or proceed with extreme caution.

What role do medications and supplements play in managing Metabolic Syndrome?

Medications and supplements can complement lifestyle changes in managing metabolic syndrome, but they are not standalone solutions.

- **Medications:** Metformin is a first-line medication that improves insulin sensitivity and reduces glucose production. GLP-1 agonists (e.g., Ozempic, Semaglutide) mimic hormones that enhance insulin secretion, promote weight loss, and offer cardiovascular benefits. These medications are often prescribed to manage specific components of metabolic syndrome, like high blood sugar and weight.
- **Supplements:** Certain supplements show promise in supporting metabolic health. Omega-3 fatty acids can reduce triglycerides and inflammation. Berberine may help regulate blood sugar and improve lipid profiles. Magnesium is crucial for glucose metabolism and blood pressure regulation. Vitamin D is linked to reduced risks of obesity and insulin resistance.

However, relying *solely* on pills without addressing lifestyle factors poses risks, including side effects, financial burden, and neglecting the underlying issues. An **integrative approach** that combines medicine with comprehensive lifestyle modifications is essential for effective and sustainable management of metabolic syndrome.

Who is most at risk for Metabolic Syndrome, and what are some early warning signs?

Certain groups are at a higher risk for developing metabolic syndrome:

- **Family History:** Individuals with a familial history of diabetes or cardiovascular disease.
- **Age:** Risk increases with age due to metabolic changes.
- **Lifestyle Choices:** Sedentary behavior, poor diet, and excessive alcohol consumption are significant contributors.
- **Gender:** Men generally have a higher risk, but post-menopausal women also see an increased risk due to hormonal changes.
- **Ethnic Groups:** Higher prevalence rates are observed in Hispanic, African American, and Native American populations, often intersected by socioeconomic factors.

Early warning signs and related conditions that act as red flags include:

- **Pre-diabetes:** Elevated blood glucose levels not yet high enough for a diabetes diagnosis.
- **Polycystic Ovary Syndrome (PCOS):** A hormonal disorder in women closely linked to insulin resistance.
- **Fatty Liver Disease (NAFLD):** Accumulation of fat in liver cells, often signaling underlying insulin resistance.
- **Waist-to-Hip Ratio:** A higher ratio indicates more dangerous abdominal fat distribution, even if overall weight seems normal.
- **Abnormal Blood Test Results:** Elevated fasting glucose, HbA1c (average blood sugar over 2-3 months), high triglycerides, and low HDL cholesterol are key indicators.

Recognizing these risk factors and early signs through regular health screenings is crucial for timely intervention.

How can one design and sustain a personal Metabolic Reset Plan effectively?

Designing and sustaining a personal metabolic reset plan requires a structured, realistic, and consistent approach:

- **Self-Assessment:** Use a "Where Do You Stand?" checklist to evaluate current body measurements (waist circumference, BMI), diet, physical activity levels, blood pressure, cholesterol, and family history. This provides a baseline and identifies risk factors.
- **Set SMART Goals:** Define Specific, Measurable, Achievable, Relevant, and Time-bound goals (e.g., "lose 5 kg in 3 months" or "exercise 30 minutes 5 times a week"). This provides clarity and motivation.
- **Structured Program (e.g., 4-Week Reset):** Gradually eliminate processed foods, sugars, and unhealthy fats; focus on whole foods; practice portion control and mindful eating; incorporate at least 150 minutes of moderate exercise weekly; and emphasize stress management.
- **Tracking Tools:** Utilize apps, journals, or devices to monitor health metrics, diet, and physical activity. This provides real-time data and enhances accountability.
- **Habit Stacking:** Link new healthy habits to existing routines (e.g., drink water after brushing teeth) to make adoption easier and more sustainable.
- **Overcoming Setbacks:** Recognize that setbacks and plateaus are normal. Introduce variety into routines, reassess goals, practice self-compassion, and seek support to break through stagnation.
- **Support Networks and Accountability:** Friends, family, coaches, or support groups provide crucial encouragement, personalized guidance, and accountability, fostering long-term adherence to lifestyle changes.
- **Consistency:** Emphasize that managing metabolic syndrome is a lifelong commitment. Incremental, consistent changes are more sustainable than drastic overhauls, leading to lasting results and improved quality of life.

16

📚 Books

1. **"Fatty Liver Diet Guide and Cookbook"** by Dr. Jonathan S. Lee*Easy-to-understand guide with diet plans, practical tips, and education for patients with NAFLD.*
2. **"The Liver Healing Diet"** by Michelle Lai, MD & Asha Kasaraneni, MD*A practical resource written by hepatologists covering lifestyle strategies to heal the liver naturally.*
3. **"Metabolic Syndrome and Liver Disease"** (Academic, Springer Series)*A more technical book for professionals connecting the dots between insulin resistance, NAFLD, and liver pathologies.*
4. **"The End of Fatty Liver Disease"** by Dr. Sandra Cabot*Holistic approach combining nutritional therapy, liver support supplements, and lifestyle changes.*

17

Articles & Journals

1. **"Global epidemiology of nonalcoholic fatty liver disease"** – *Nature Reviews Gastroenterology & Hepatology (2023)*https://www.nature.com/articles/s41575-023-00758-3
2. **"Nonalcoholic fatty liver disease: A practical guide"** – *American Family Physician,* 2022https://www.aafp.org
3. **"Association of NAFLD with Metabolic Syndrome and Type 2 Diabetes"** – *Diabetes & Metabolic Syndrome: Clinical Research & Reviews (2021)*
4. **"Treatment of NAFLD: Current guidelines and emerging therapies"** – *Journal of Hepatology (2022)*
5. **"Fatty Liver Disease: A Growing Public Health Concern"** – *BMJ,* 2023 https://www.bmj.com

18

Websites & Clinical Guidelines

For Patients

- **Liver Foundation (Australia)***Patient-friendly education, support, and resources for Australians with liver conditions.*
- **American Liver Foundation***Fact sheets, videos, and tools for managing NAFLD and NASH.*
- **British Liver Trust***Excellent visual guides and risk assessment tools for fatty liver.*

For Clinicians

- **EASL Clinical Practice Guidelines** – European Association for the Study of the Liver*Widely accepted diagnostic and treatment guidelines for NAFLD/-NASH.*
- **UpToDate (Subscription)***Authoritative clinical reference on NAFLD pathophysiology, workup, and management.*
- **Therapeutic Guidelines (eTG Australia)***Australian clinical treatment pathways related to metabolic syndrome and liver function.*

www.ingramcontent.com/pod-product-compliance
Lightning Source LLC
LaVergne TN
LVHW090425210926
848480LV00002B/690
* 9 7 9 8 2 3 2 4 4 7 5 6 4 *